Guidelines on Patient Care in Radiography

Christine Gunn TDCR
Formerly Deputy Principal,
Derbyshire Royal Infirmary School of Radiography

Christine S. Jackson TDCR DipAdEd
Principal,
Hogarth School of Radiotherapy,
Nottingham

SECOND EDITION

CHURCHILL LIVINGSTONE
EDINBURGH LONDON MELBOURNE NEW YORK AND TOKYO 1991

CHURCHILL LIVINGSTONE
Medical Division of Longman Group UK Limited

Distributed in the United States of America by Churchill
Livingstone Inc., 1560 Broadway, New York, N.Y. 10036,
and by associated companies, branches and representatives
throughout the world.

First edition 1982
Second edition 1991

ISBN 0-443-04391-4

British Library Cataloguing in Publication Data

Gunn, Christine
  Guidelines on patient care in radiography. — 2nd. ed.
  1. Medicine. Radiology
  I. Title II. Jackson, Christine S.
  616.0757

Library of Congress Cataloging in Publication Data

Gunn, Christine.
  Guidelines on patient care in radiography/Christine Gunn,
Christine S. Jackson. — 2nd ed.
    p. cm.
  Includes index.
  ISBN 0-443-04391-4
  1. Radiography, Medical. 2. Radiotherapy. 3. Radiologic technologists.
  4. Nursing. I. Jackson, Christine S. II. Title.
    [DNLM: 1. Hospital Departments — organization & administration —
  handbooks. 2. Patients — handbooks. 3. Radiography — handbooks.
  4. Radiotherapy — handbooks. WN 39 G976g]
  RC78.G86 1991
  616.07′572 — dc20
  DNLM/DLC   90-15100
  for Library of Congress   CIP

Produced by Longman Singapore Publishers (Pte) Ltd.
Printed in Singapore

Guidelines on Patient Care in Radiography

For Churchill Livingstone:
Publisher: Mary Law
Project Editor: Dinah Thom
Design: Design Resources Unit
Production: Nancy Henry
Sales Promotion Executive: Marion Pollock

Preface

This book was written as a precise reference guide to the care of the patient in the Imaging and Radiotherapy departments.

Our aim is to provide essential information which may be of use, not only to student radiographers and radiographers but also to X-ray and Radiotherapy nurses and other paramedical staff having contact with patients.

We anticipate that student radiographers will use the guide alongside more detailed texts which, together with the relevant practical experience, will help to provide the student radiographer with a sound basis on which to develop a high standard of patient care.

The 25 chapters contain information on all aspects of patient care. At the beginning of each chapter, an introduction outlines the reasons why the information which follows has been included. Since writing the first edition new techniques, contrast agents, drug classifications, and legislation have been introduced and computers are more frequently used. We have updated the original information on inflammation and infection and have incorporated the care of the patient with HIV infection. It is difficult to know how much information is necessary (or unnecessary) and we have tried to produce a book which achieves a balance between a purely factual notebook and a detailed textbook.

We would like to thank the College of Radiographers for giving us permission to use abstracts from Examiners' comments, College Guidelines and the Code of Professional Conduct.

The following people have read parts of the manuscripts and offered advice and professional comment: Pam Cox, Joyce Davidson, Gary Ferguson, Mike Gordon, Donald Graham, Don Gunn, Tim Heath, Lynn Hicks, Andrew Loveridge, Dave Mackay, Sub-

Officer Myers, Alan Riddoch, Mary Smith, Philip Thornhill, Helen
Turner, Stuart Whitley. Without their help this new edition would
not have been possible.

1991   C.G.
                                                         C.S.J.

Contents

1. Departmental organisation and procedure

INTRODUCTION

The aim of this section is to provide the student radiographer with information regarding general departmental procedures. It is important that the student is aware that the practical running of hospital departments requires an efficient hospital team of which they have become a member. Emphasis must be placed on gaining practical experience within their own departments and the guidelines set out in this chapter should help the student to have an understanding of departmental organisation and the importance of record keeping.

At the end of this section are notes concerning medico-legal aspects of hospital administration and current management structures.

Whilst we feel that to burden students with complicated legal procedures and laws is unnecessary, nevertheless a basic appreciation of medico-legal aspects regarding hospital personnel and patients in the department should be within the capabilities of student radiographers.

WAITING AREAS

When planning waiting areas the following points should be considered:

  Sufficient area to accommodate patients and 'friends'
  Separate areas for children/badly injured/ward patients
  Sufficient comfortable chairs, at different heights, and small tables
  Well ventilated, no draughts, suitable temperature
  Pleasant decor and good lighting

Clean magazines, goldfish, piped music and plants may be available

Toys for children (washable — to reduce the likelihood of infection)

Toilet facilities — adjacent and well signposted

Non-slip floors

Ramps used instead of steps

Fire exits clearly marked

Refreshments available or instructions where they can be obtained

Receptionist available to assist the patients.

CHANGING ROOMS

Should have:
  A fixed chair or seat
  Hooks for clothes
  A mirror
  Locks which can be opened from the outside in an emergency
  Enough space for a wheelchair
  Lockers available for clothing and valuables.

TOILETS

Should have:
  Non-slip floors
  Safety rails
  A bell for emergency use
  Hand washing facilities
  Paper towels or warm air driers
They should be well lit and large enough for a wheelchair to be positioned next to the toilet.

APPOINTMENT SYSTEMS

Required to:
  Minimise patient waiting time
  Ensure full use of staff and equipment
When booking an appointment —
  Avoid overbooking
  Remember to leave room for emergencies

Ask the patient to inform the department if they are unable to attend

For In Patients avoid

Meal times

Doctors ward rounds

Drug administration rounds

Visiting time

For Out Patients consider

The distance the patient has to travel and the time it may take

Use of hostel accommodation for radiotherapy patients

If the patient is on 'shift work'

If the patient has dependants (young children, etc.)

If the appointment can be arranged to coincide with other hospital visits

If an ambulance will be required

If an ambulance escort will be required

Any clinical features e.g. a strict schedule is required for diabetic patients

DIAGNOSTIC X-RAY EXAMINATION REQUEST FORMS

Ideally these should give the following information:

Patient details

Full name

Address

Hospital registration number

Age/date of birth

X-ray number

Occupation

Sex

Married/single/widowed

Method of transport from the ward e.g. if a trolley is required

Ward/Out patient

Record answer to, 'Are you, or might you be pregnant?'

Date of last menstrual period if required

Date and place of previous radiographs

Departmental information

Radiographic examination requested

Doctor's signature/personal computer code authorisation

Consultant in charge of the case
Any clinical features/diagnosis
If the patient is, or may be, pregnant and the referring clinician and/or radiologist states the examination must not go ahead. Record that the procedure has been followed
Number of films for reporting
Radiographer's signature
Exposure factors used
Type, dose, batch number and time of injection of contrast agent if used
Space for the radiologist's report

The above information is required to ensure that the correct patient is radiographed and any previous radiographs/reports can be obtained. The person referring the patient and the radiographer responsible for the radiographs can be contacted if necessary.

PATIENT CASE HISTORY — RADIOTHERAPY AND ONCOLOGY

Patient identified by referring hospital number
Radiotherapy — oncology file opened and number assigned
Case number and history may be colour coded to show year treatment commenced
Patient data — it is vital to give as much personal detail as possible for accurate call up.
Radiotherapy request form
Patient treatment details
Test results
Consent form

Computerisation of patients' notes within a health district allows cross-linked access with peripheral clinics.
Provides for accurate transfer of patient data
Rapid booking of appointment times etc.

Storage of patient's case history

Hard copy notes create storage problems, especially long term notes.
Microfiche storage — reduces bulk storage problems but expensive and time consuming to set up.
Data Base systems — useful for research purposes. Expensive and time consuming to set up.

Departments may have a policy for destruction of some patients notes (i.e. 3 years after death).

RADIOTHERAPY PRESCRIPTIONS

Ideally they should give the following information:

Patient details

Full name
Hospital number
Diagnosis
In/Out patient
Prescribing consultant and signature

Treatment details

Treatment machine
Beam energy/modality
Focus to skin distance
Field sizes
Position of fields
Beam direction devices
Wedges
Compensators
Treatment plan
Target dose
Skin dose
Applied dose
Special instructions e.g. blood counts to be undertaken
Information recorded daily by the radiographer during treatment
Summary of treatment on completion

DEPARTMENTAL STATISTICS

Diagnostic

Records are kept concerning:
    Patient attendances — In/Out patients
    The number of radiographic examinations undertaken
    The number of Körner units
Körner units are based on the cost of an examination and are a

method of comparing different departments. The code given depends on the type of examination and is divided into 6 groups

Group	Numbered from	Example examination
A	100	Extremities
B	200	Ultrasound, Skull
C	300	Computed tomography
D	400	Excretion urography
E	500	Lymphangiography, Lumbar radiculography
F	600	Magnetic resonance imaging

There is no extra weighting for theatre, mobile work etc.
The statistics are used for:
  Manpower planning
  Utilisation of rooms
  Regional data.
Records are kept for 8 years after the conclusion of treatment except for:
  Obstetric records – 25 years
  Mentally disordered – 20 years
  Children – until they reach the age of 25 or 8 years after the last entry

Radiotherapy

Statistics are kept annually concerning:
  Number of new cases
  Total number of treated cases
  Number of attendances
  Number of radiation exposures
  Number of specialist exposures (total body irradiation, hemibody irradiation)
  Number of specialist treatments (using unsealed radionuclides, afterloading units)

Treatment planning

Similar figures are required for:
  Simulator work
  Computerised tomography planning
  Computer planning

Treatment unit statistics

To include:
Patient numbers per month
In patients/Out patients
Running up procedures
Required to enable a quantifiable machine activity analysis to be provided.

Körner manpower

Sickness and absence statistics
Staffing levels — starters and leavers

COMPUTERISATION OF IMAGING DEPARTMENTS

Computerisation is taking place in many areas of the health service.

Advantages

Ease of administration
Appointments can be booked quickly
Labels/bar codes/appointment letters automatically produced
Reports can be generated
Films can be traced
Statistics can be generated e.g.
Körner units
Patient attendances
Types of examination/treatment
Workload per room
Cost breakdown and stock keeping of e.g.
Films
Chemicals
Contrast agents

Disadvantages

1 Initially very expensive to set up
2 Unauthorised access must not be possible

To prevent this

Passwords are issued; these control the amount of information which can be obtained from/fed into the system; the number of levels will depend on the size of the system.

For example, depending on the type of password the user may do one of the following:

Look up a minimum amount of information e.g. patients' names and addresses

Add a limited amount of information e.g. booking appointments

See a patient's notes e.g. prior to treatment

Add to a patient's notes e.g. generate an imaging request form.

The owner of the password is legally responsible for it and should not disclose it to anyone else.

To prevent unauthorised use, passwords are changed at regular intervals e.g. every 6 months.

3 The Data Protection Act must be followed

This covers all personal information stored on a computer and is designed to protect an individual from unauthorised disclosure of information.

Therefore:

All personal data and its use must be registered

The person about whom the data is held is entitled to know about it

The user must observe the principles of the Act

NB. The Data Protection Act only applies to computer records and not to handwritten notes.

It is the user and not the data that must be registered.

4 Loss of information due to electricity failure etc.

To prevent this, the computer system is 'backed up' throughout the day and at night.

This may be done on 8 mm video tape.

A duplicate copy of all information is kept in a separate building.

Storage of radiographs

Each radiograph should give the following information (preferably photographed on)

Patient's name

Hospital

The date the radiographic examination was undertaken

An anatomical marker

Patient identification number

Radiographs are stored in paper envelopes which carry details of
  Patient's name
  X-ray number
  The radiographic examinations which have been performed
Radiographs can be filed under
  X-ray registration number
  The date of birth of the patient
  The patient's name (in alphabetical order)
Radiographs should be stored
  Away from direct heat
  Away from damp
  In an area of constant temperature

ORGANISATION OF THE NATIONAL HEALTH SERVICE

1983–4
Griffiths Report recommendations to the Government, a change in
Health Service management
The report outlined definite lines of responsibility and the creation
of General Manager posts

1989
Publication of the White Paper 'Working for Patients'
Two prime objectives
  Better health care and greater choice
  Greater rewards for hospital workers who successfully respond to
  local needs
Key measures include
  Allowing hospitals to apply for self-governing status
  Creation of new consultant posts
  Allowing General Practitioner practices to apply for their own
  budgets
  Ensuring effective monitoring of resources by setting up a
  Medical Audit System
  Basis for the National Health Service and Community Care Act
  1990

MEDICO-LEGAL ASPECTS

Medical ethics

A set of moral values and principles of conduct for professionals
working with patients

Ethical responsibilities include

Confidentiality
Not revealing diagnoses of patients
Patient consent obtained, when required
Code of professional conduct for radiographers should be followed
   With reference to
   Work
   Relationships with patients
   Relationships with colleagues

Informed consent

Written consent required for:
   Investigations which require a general anaesthetic
   Procedures which may involve a special risk
Patients given a full explanation of the procedure, in terms they can understand.

Problems with obtaining consent

Lack of understanding — confusion, illness, senility
Age, if under 18
Patient already sedated
Patient may refuse and has the right to refuse without censure

Accidents in an imaging or radiotherapy department

Injury to patients may be caused by:
Imaging equipment/treatment units
Hazards
   mechanical
   radiation
   electrical
Accessory equipment
Hazards arising from use of:
   couch
   applicators or cones
   cassettes, grids
   patient transport
Departmental
   Poor lighting
   Incorrect storage
   Poor repair of buildings, internal or external

Patient care procedures
Following an accident or injury to a patient
  Give appropriate first aid
  Report to head of department immediately
  Inform the Medical Officer
  Write up accident and occurrence report

Major accident (incident) procedure

Major accident — more than 15 casualties
Determined by first senior officer on the scene
Head of Department informed of
  Type and extent of the accident
  Approximate number of casualties
  Estimated time of arrival
Depending on the time of day, plan may involve
  Rescheduling booked appointments
  Allocation of staff and rooms
  Recalling mobile imaging unit
  Liaison with accident and emergency with regard to patient
  identity
All staff should have adequate breaks

HEALTH AND SAFETY AT WORK ACT

Instituted in 1974
Applies to all persons at work (except domestic employees in
private households)
Principal objectives
  To involve all staff at the work place and to create an awareness
  of the importance of achieving a high standard of health and
  safety
  It is the duty of everyone to take reasonable care for health and
  safety.

Crown immunity was removed from Health Service premises in
February 1987
The Health Service can now be prosecuted under the Health and
Safety at Work Act
Employers' duties include
  Providing policies for safe working practices
  Consulting Health and Safety Representatives and establishing
  the Safety Committee

Providing information on:
    training
    welfare
    safety policies

The College of Radiographers produces guidelines to assist radiographers
For example:

Guidelines for implementation of ASP8 Exposure to ionising radiation of pregnant women: Advice on the diagnostic exposure of women who are, or who may be, pregnant (1986)
Covers
The procedure to be followed for diagnostic examinations of women of reproductive capacity.

Guidelines for radiographers working with patients diagnosed as suffering from, or suspected of suffering from, HIV (AIDS) (1987)
Covers
Professional responsibility of radiographers
Patient care
Health Service who are HIV antibody positive
Test for HIV virus.

Control of infection protocol (1987)
Covers
Informing staff
Care of cuts and abrasions
A suggested departmental protocol

RIDDOR (1985)   (Reporting of Injuries, Disease and Dangerous Occurrences Regulations)

This enables the Health and Safety Executive (HSE) to monitor and enforce safety regulations

Following an accident or occurrence, the RIDDOR system enables the information to be passed to the HSE via NHS administration.

COSHH REGULATIONS   (Control of substances hazardous to health)

Specific extension to duties of the employer (1st October 1989)

Basic principle

Risk to health rising from working with hazardous substances must be assessed

Substances covered by COSHH include

Microbiological substances

Carcinogenic teratogenic substances (excluding ionising radiations)

Drugs and pharmaceuticals (where there is a hazard to staff)

Regulations cover

Prevention and control of exposure

Testing and monitoring of exposure

Health surveillance

Information, instruction and training

COSHH regulations do not cover use of asbestos, lead or ionising radiations for which separate legislation exists.

PROFESSIONAL ATTITUDES

The College of Radiographers has produced a Code of Professional Conduct for Radiographers. Students should be aware of the contents of the document and ensure that they follow the Code.

Radiographers should:

Offer the best possible service to patients

Keep the radiation dose as low as possible

Act in a manner to justify public trust and confidence.

With reference to:

Patients

Treat as individuals with rights and needs

Treat with dignity and respect

Care for physical and psychological needs

Avoid abuse of patients or property

Ensure well being and interests of patients are safeguarded

Hold in confidence any information obtained.

Work

Comply with the law of the land

Be accountable for their work

Only accept authorised requests for examinations or treatment

Sustain and improve knowledge and professional competence

Request additional training/support if required

Make known to the appropriate authority any relevant conscientious objection held

Ensure professional responsibilities and standards are not influenced by religion, sex, race, nationality, party politics, social or economic status or a patient's health problems

Refuse any gift, favour or hospitality which may be interpreted as seeking preferential treatment

Avoid advertising to encourage the sale of commercial products.

Other staff

Accept responsibility for the development of professional competence

Be aware of workloads of others and assist where necessary

Adopt safe working practices

Co-operate with others

Report unethical conduct.

2. Hygiene

INTRODUCTION

It is essential that student radiographers understand and practise the rules relating to hygiene with regard to themselves, their patients and the working environment.

A high standard of hygiene is expected from every member of staff in the hospital and the following section is intended to help the student to develop a common sense approach to hygiene standards.

To ensure that cross-infection is kept to a minimum the following points should be considered —

Personal

Uniform coats should
>Be clean and changed when necessary
>Cover clothing
>Only be worn inside the hospital
>Be of the correct length and not too tight

Protective gowns should be worn in theatre and when handling an infectious patient

Footwear
>Shoes should be comfortable and in good repair
>Shoes should be quiet, safe, protective and only worn inside the hospital
>Socks/tights should be clean
>Special shoes should be worn in the operating theatre.

Hair should be
>Either short or tied back
>Clean and tidy
>Covered completely in the operating theatre

15

Diet
  Should be well balanced
  Regular meals should be taken
  Regular bowel habits are to be encouraged
  Care should be taken with regard to dental hygiene
Bathing
  Reduces infection
  Is refreshing and relaxing
In general
  Finger nails, short, clean, with no nail varnish
  If watches and jewellery are worn, care should be taken to ensure
  that there are no sharp edges which could scratch a patient
  Face masks should be worn when necessary
  Cuts on hands should be covered with waterproof dressings
  Hands must be washed after handling patients/dressings/bedpans/
  urinals/catheters/soiled instruments etc.

Patient

Clean gowns/bed linen/cubicles/X-ray room/treatment room
Disposable materials and equipment used e.g. syringes/needles/
drinking receptacles/denture holders/bedpans
Hand washing facilities must be available

Equipment

Kept socially clean
Special care with equipment for use in the operating theatre
Use of washable items e.g. foam pads/covers for sandbags and bolus
bags
Sterile equipment used for aseptic procedures
Use of covered receptacles for used dressings
Infected material should be disposed of in sealed, colour coded bags

Department

Kept socially clean/vacuumed to prevent dust
Good ventilation/air conditioning — checked regularly to avoid
spread of disease causing pathogens e.g. Legionella
Equipment kept in cupboards and so free from dust
Adequate washing facilities should be available
'Clean' and 'dirty' examinations kept separate

Special areas reserved for surgical trolley setting
Toilet facilities checked and cleaned regularly
Hand washing facilities — hot water temperature 60°C at the
cylinder and not less than 50°C at the tap to reduce risk of
Legionella contamination
Separate hot water taps carry a temperature warning notice
Department procedures for dealing with patients who are likely to
be suffering from infection, see Chapter 6 (Inflammation and
infection)

3. Management of patients and patient psychology

INTRODUCTION

Throughout the training period and following on to the post qualification period, radiographers will experience a variety of patient personalities and patients with special difficulties needing extra attention.

Students will quickly be confronted by a variety of problems which will need patience and a lot of common sense. The way in which people respond towards patients depends a great deal on their own personality but with the practical guidelines of this chapter, combined with the experiences learnt in the department the student should develop both a psychological and practical competence for handling patients.

GENERAL PATIENT PSYCHOLOGY

Treat all patients with courtesy and respect
Refer to patients by name
Be polite, efficient and sympathetic
Be aware of emotional problems connected with
  Illness
  Treatment/examination procedures
  Hospitals
  Their self-esteem, which may be low
  Loss of individuality due to the loss of job,
  finance, status etc.
Be careful when coping with
  Relatives
  Racial problems in an interracial society
Be aware of physical problems associated with
  Illness

Age
Low level of intelligence

COMMUNICATING WITH THE PATIENT

Do we always do our best to communicate with and understand our patients' needs?
Do we:
Always give the patient enough time
Face the patient squarely when talking or listening
Keep good eye contact, showing interest and concern
Create the opportunity for personal communication by adopting a natural stance (not with arms folded)
Try to be at the same eye level as the patient, standing above a seated patient will make him feel awkward
Bring comfort to a distressed patient by touching him — physical contact brings a person closer to another but be aware if this is not acceptable
Encourage new students, not accustomed to physical patient contact, to help with the lifting of patients
Share a sense of humour with our patients
Encourage patients to talk of their fears and problems by asking 'open ended' questions e.g. 'How are you managing at home when the treatment is making you tired?'
If the answer to these questions is yes, then you care for your patient.

The psychological impact of illness/cancer

The state of being in good health is something we all take for granted. Not until this state changes, do we appreciate that our lifestyle depends upon continuing good health.

What problems do we have to face when our health takes a change for the worse?

What anxieties are our patients suffering when they take their first step into the imaging or radiotherapy departments?

Put yourself in their place.

General illness

What is wrong with me?
Do you know my diagnosis?
Am I going to get better?
Will I suffer any pain — with the illness
                          with the investigations?

Will I look any different?
Will I feel any different?
Why has it happened to me?
Will you answer all my questions?
Will you think of me as an individual in my own right?
Will I remember all of your instructions?
Will you think that I am stupid if I forget what you have told me?
Will I have to come again?

Cancer patients

Why has it happened to me?
Where have I got it from?
Have I really got cancer?
When am I going to die?
Will I feel any pain?
Why does the operation scar look so ugly?
Do I look ugly to you?
Why do some people avoid my questions?
Why have I heard so many conflicting stories about radiotherapy?
Will it burn my skin?
Will it burn me inside?
Will I feel sick?
Will my hair fall out?
Will the radiation make me sterile?
Will I become radioactive?
Will I remember all my instructions?
When will I feel better?
Why was Mrs X so ill after her treatment?
Will I have to come back for some more treatment?
Why do I have to have all these tests and investigations?
Is it true that cancer is curable?
Could I be one of the lucky ones?
Shall I start planning for the future?

General problems

Can I cope with all this?
Who will look after my children, wife, husband, parents, animals?
Should I make a will?
Who will pay the bills?
Who will do the shopping?
Who will service the car?
Will I be able to drive?

Who will explain about the tablets which I am taking?
What will I tell my family and friends?
When can I start work again?
Will I have a job to return to?
Why have people started to treat me differently?
Am I of any use?
Will my life ever be the same?
Do you now see what 'Care of the patient' is all about?

Role of patient support worker in imaging or radiotherapy departments

Before treatment or imaging starts:
   Give patient an opportunity to voice fears
   Encourage the asking of questions
   Give accurate and comprehensive information — verbal and written
   Reinforce information given by doctors
   Give emotional support

Care and support for the radiographer

Caring for, and supporting, patients can be
emotionally as well as physically demanding
It is important to recognise that radiographers
may, at times, require support because of the
stress and demands of the job
It can be beneficial to talk over your concerns
and worries
The following hospital personnel can provide
support if required:
Patient support worker/counsellor
Radiotherapy social worker
Nursing and medical staff — Occupational Health

Provision of care for terminally ill patients

Care of the patient at home

Should the patient wish it and relatives are able to cope
Benefits include
Familiar surroundings
Greater freedom
Relatively normal life-style, privacy

Family and friends more accessible
Nursing care is not too clinical
Support of day care service if required — nursing, paramedical service, social workers, volunteer groups, chaplain services
Development of night care services in progress
Problems
Fear of medical assistance not immediately available
Extra burden on family.

Hospital/continuing care unit

Aims of hospice care

To provide medical care and pain relief
To relieve relatives of some of the care
To develop community services for the terminally ill
Bereavement counselling
Development of hospital support teams — advising staff on general wards.
Benefits of hospice care
Minimum clinical intrusion, maximum clinical support
Advanced symptom control techniques/individually designed care
Nurse to patient ratio — can be 1:1
Attention to detail — food requirements etc.
Support for relatives.
Disadvantages
Fear of attending special unit
Distance from home
Isolation from family
Separate hospices required for patients with chronic illnesses, children's hospices.

Hearing impaired patients

Take special care when checking their identity
Make a note of their disability on the request form/treatment sheet
Use clear, slow speech
Face the patient as they may be able to lip read
Use sign language/written instructions
Always fetch a patient from the waiting area
Touch patients to gain their attention if necessary
Check the understanding of instructions by asking the patient to repeat them
Avoid unnecessary chatter which may confuse the patient

Avoid hazards e.g. approaching trolleys
Ensure the patient understands when they can leave
Check transport details
Never shout at the patient
Return hearing aids promptly (if they have been removed during
the treatment/examination).

Visually handicapped patients

Respect their independence
Note the disability on request form/treatment sheet
Carefully guide the patient, avoiding obstacles, ask the person how
they like to be guided e.g. by holding your arm or touching your
shoulder
Inform the patient about the length of corridors/of any steps/if the
route is either flat or sloping/if doors open inwards or outwards
Explain procedures carefully including any noises e.g. tomographic
equipment/treatment machine noise
Indicate the length of time they will be required to wait
Care with the guide dog
If you leave the room, inform the patient
If the patient has to wait e.g. for an ambulance, arrange for a mem-
ber of staff to speak to the patient at regular intervals to ensure he
is all right.

Patient with English language difficulties

Extra care when checking their identity
Clear, simple language if some English is understood
Possible use of an interpreter e.g. a member of staff or a relative
to explain instructions
Use sign language/demonstrate/cue cards
Give written instructions for future examinations/treatments.

Care of children

Care required depends on age of child and quality of initial prepara-
tion for treatment/investigation in paediatric clinic
Staff numbers kept to a minimum but take extra care over con-
tinuity of staff
Speak directly to the child and listen to him
Answer questions truthfully
Avoid undue waiting

Friendly approach with extra patience
Try to win the child's confidence
Have pictures and toys available.
Do not exclude parents as good liaison is important — explanation of possible side effects
In an imaging department use discretion regarding the presence of parents during the examination
Consider demonstrating on the parents (do not irradiate)
Careful use of restraining/immobilisation devices
Encourage child to look forward to future examinations/treatments
Consider:
    Children's waiting areas
    Play equipment
    Safety aspects
Use sedation for unco-operative child only as a last resort.

Care of the less able elderly patients

An increasing proportion of the population is 65 or over.
Commonest causes of death are:
    Ischaemic heart disease
    Stroke
    Respiratory disease including cancer
    Cancer of the digestive tract
Care of the elderly patient is becoming an increasing part of the radiographer's workload
Do not have preconceived ideas of what an elderly patient will be like.

Less able elderly

Avoid patronising the patient
Consider whether extra time is needed
Be aware of reduced short-term memory
Be aware and allow for any physical disabilities
Involvement of younger relations should the patient so wish

Diseases occurring with increasing age

Alzheimer's disease
Parkinson's disease

Hemiplegic (patient is paralysed down one side)

Exercise care when lifting the patient
Special care with the paralysed side
Remove objects from the table top/treatment couch to prevent injury
Ensure limbs are on the trolley/table and are not under the patient

An unconscious patient

If possible radiograph/treat when the department is not busy
Have suction and oxygen equipment available
The emergency tray should be available
Observe the patient to ensure that:
    A clear airway is maintained
    There is no change in the skin colour
    The pulse and respiration rates are taken and recorded
Any change in condition should be reported
Speed and adaptation of technique is required
Do not leave unattended
Return to the ward/accident and emergency department with an escort

Care of patient valuables

Discourage patients from bringing valuables and excess amounts of money into the hospital
Provision of a safe storage place — under lock and key
Patient and radiographer should check the contents
Patient should be issued with a receipt
Return valuables to the patient promptly
Ensure the patient signs for their return

An aggressive patient

Be tactful and honest
Try to keep calm
Do not retaliate
Try to defuse the situation
Try to find the reason e.g. waiting time, fear etc.
Protect yourself and others.

4. Care of the unconscious and anaesthetised patient

INTRODUCTION

During the course of their work student radiographers will come into contact with unconscious and anaesthetised patients. In the diagnostic department patients may be seen directly after a major accident, or may require a general anaesthetic for more specialised examinations.

In the radiotherapy department, anaesthetised patients with carcinoma of the cervix/uterus will require check radiographs for positioning and dosage calculations prior to caesium insertion (afterloading technique).

Young, unco-operative children may require general anaesthetic in order to induce narcosis for treatment purposes.

Student radiographers should be aware of how to care for these patients and be familiar with any complications which may occur.

POSSIBLE CAUSES OF UNCONSCIOUSNESS

General anaesthetic
Brain tumour
Cardiac arrest
Cerebrovascular accident
Concussion
Diabetic coma
Drowning
Drug overdose
Epileptic fit
Fainting
Haemorrhage
Insulin coma
Poisoning.

CARE OF THE UNCONSCIOUS PATIENT

Airway

Check for obstruction which may be due to vomit, false teeth etc.
If the patient is supine, lower jaw is held forward
An artificial airway may be inserted
Expired air resuscitation may be administered if required

Pulse

Check heart beat, note — rate, strength, regularity
Administer cardiac massage if required.

Patient position

Place in the recovery position — unless contraindicated
Ensure the patient is kept warm and has privacy
Ensure plenty of fresh air.

Haemorrhage

Check for bleeding — treat as necessary
Check skin colour/respiratory rate/any change in the level of consciousness.

General

Reassure the patient — hearing is the first sense to return
Give nothing by mouth
Do not leave the patient unattended
Check equipment is functioning correctly e.g. infusion sets/oxygen etc.

UNCONSCIOUS PATIENTS IN THE X-RAY DEPARTMENT

Patients in an accident and emergency department

Speed is essential when dealing with the patient
Do not keep the patient waiting
Have cassettes and X-ray equipment ready
Plan the order in which the radiographs are taken — to prevent

undue movement of the patient e.g. all lateral projections exposed
in succession
Double check the patient's identity
Do not leave the patient unattended.

OPERATING THEATRE PROCEDURE

Ensure mobile X-ray unit/cassettes cleaned e.g. with suitable
disinfectant
Wash hands and cover cuts with waterproof dressing
Correct clothing, mask, cap, gown, theatre shoes worn by
radiographer
Put on lead rubber apron and radiation monitoring badge.
Check that it is the correct patient
Care taken not to contaminate sterile areas
Cover the X-ray tube head before placing over sterile field
Ask anaesthetist to control patient's respiration during exposure
Take and return films quickly.

After the operation

Dispose of theatre clothing
Clean mobile X-ray unit
Check identity of films.

UNCONSCIOUS PATIENTS IN THE RADIOTHERAPY DEPARTMENT

Young children are usually the only patients to be anaesthetised
under the radiographer's care.

These are young children who are totally unco-operative during
treatment.

A fast acting drug is needed to induce narcosis.

Throughout the treatment period there should be liaison with:
The radiotherapist
Department of anaesthetics
Ward staff (if child is an In patient)
Ambulance department
The parents
Ensure that:
Instructions are given about meal arrangements
Appointment time given to suit all involved in the procedure,

if possible the same time each day; the first appointment in the morning is often the most suitable
Oxygen, suction and emergency drugs are available
Treatment given as quickly as possible
Provision for monitoring the heart rate during treatment is made
Quiet room for recovery period is available.

Other patients under anaesthetic include:

Females with carcinoma cervix/uterus prior to caesium insertion (afterloading)
Patient with radioactive implants e.g. tongue, buccal mucosal.
These patients require check radiographs for positioning and dosage calculations.

PATIENTS FOR GENERAL ANAESTHETIC

Check

Identity bracelet (on either the arm or leg)
Correct notes and radiographs have arrived with the patient
Dentures removed, mouth clean
Procedure has been explained
Consent form signed
Correct clothing worn
Jewellery removed, wedding ring taped, nail varnish and dentures removed

Premedication

Action

Achieves sedation
Depresses reflex activity
Inhibits bronchial and salivary secretions.

Drugs used

Papaveretum
Pethidine
Haloperidol.

Sedated patients

Must not be left alone
Trolley should have cot sides up
Patient may require careful restraining.

General anaesthesia

Definition — absence of sensation.
Must produce:
Narcosis (deep sleep)
Muscle relaxation
Analgesia.

Method

Intravenous injection of rapidly acting agent such as thiopentone
sodium followed by inhalation of nitrous oxide and oxygen.

During the Induction of an anaesthetic

Staff should be available and remain quiet

Where necessary

Assist with the intravenous injection
Check pulse and blood pressure
Pass drugs and instruments to the anaesthetist

After anaesthesia

Patient placed in recovery room if available
Oxygen, suction, emergency drugs should be available.

CARE OF THE ANAESTHETISED PATIENT

Airway

Artificial airway may be in the patient's mouth
If the patient is lying supine, hold the lower jaw forward
Check for any obstruction of the airway e.g. due to vomit, blood
or mucus.

Patient position

Recovery position unless contraindicated
Check limbs are on the trolley and not trapped underneath the patient
Ensure patient is warm and away from bright lights and noise.

Skin

If the skin becomes cyanosed
   Check the patient's airway
   Oxygen may be required
   Send for medical aid.

Observations

Check and record blood pressure, pulse, temperature and respiration every 15 minutes
Report any changes
Check skin colour, report any changes.

Intravenous infusions and drainage tubes

Check that infusions are working and that the tubing is not kinked or trapped.

Operation/injection site

Check every 15 minutes for
   Haemorrhage
   Haematoma
   Oedema.

Complications of general anaesthesia

Airway obstruction
Vomiting
Restlessness
Haemorrhage
Shock
Cardiac arrest
Respiratory failure.

5. Transportation of patients

INTRODUCTION

It is necessary when moving/lifting patients to adopt a technique which is safe for the patient and can be carried out without strain to the staff. For staff, the most important aspect is the problem of placing undue strain on the spinal column.

Prior to lifting

Staff should ensure that:
It is safe to lift the patient — injury may contraindicate
There are enough staff available to lift
The patient is informed
Jewellery is removed, nails are checked — care not to scratch the patient
Drips and catheters are protected
The method of lifting is planned.

PATIENTS ON TROLLEYS

NB. Patients with fractured (or suspected fractured) spines must not be moved from the trolley, except when supervised by a medical officer.

Whilst waiting

Ensure the cot sides are up
Position the trolley so that it does not cause an obstruction
Trolley should be moved by 2 members of staff
Ensure the patient is warm and away from draughts.

Before lifting the patient from trolley to X-ray table or treatment couch

Give explanation and reassurance to the patient
Ensure trolley and couch locks are on
Release cot sides
Obtain enough assistance, 3 people to lift
Check there are no obstacles in the way
Ensure the X-ray tube head is not above the table/couch
Note the position of any urinary drainage bags, intravenous infusions, fractures, wounds.
Explain the procedure to the patient
Stand in a line by the trolley
If possible, fold the patient's arms over their chest
Lifters place their arms under the patient
Ensure patient's head, buttocks and legs are supported
Bend knees, back straight — lift
Patient is supported close to the lifter's body
Together walk to the table
Keeping back straight, bending legs
Gently lower the patient into the correct position on the couch
Check that the patient's limbs are not trapped
Check that tubing is not trapped and is functioning e.g. urinary drainage bags.

Advantages of a trolley

Stable and rigid
Area for patient's clothing
Area for oxygen cylinder and column to support infusion bags or bottles
Cot sides are available
Can be locked into position
Adjustable back rest sometimes available
Patient can be radiographed on trolleys with radiolucent tops.

PATIENTS ON STRETCHERS AND POLES

Canvas stretcher with 2 wooden/metal poles which slip into the canvas
Patient placed on the canvas, on a trolley, and wheeled to the department.

Poles inserted in the sides of the canvas
Spreader placed between the poles to give the canvas rigidity
2 or 4 people required to lift
Explain procedure to the patient
Firmly grip the pole
Keeping back straight, lift the patient
Lower the patient gently onto the table
Care that infusions, drains, catheters are not dislodged
Remove poles.

Advantages of the canvas

Cheap
Easy to use
Patient can be radiographed/treated on the canvas
Easier to lift heavy patients

Special considerations when radiographing a patient with radioactive sources in situ

Make a different appointment time from other patients
Do not keep the patient waiting
Mobile protective screens can be used
Minimum time spent by the staff next to the patient's trolley
Allow nurse to attend to the care of the patient
Have the X-ray equipment ready
Return the patient to the ward as soon as possible

AIRPAL

Designed on a hovercraft principle
Patient placed on a mattress with a perforated base
Patient is secured with restraint straps
Mattress is inflated with air
The air is forced out of the base of the mattress forming a cushion of air
A friction-free surface is formed by the air
Patient is slid onto the table
The mattress is deflated.

PATIENT IN A WHEELCHAIR

Place the chair at the side of the treatment couch/table
Apply brakes

Explain the procedure to the patient
Remove the footrest
Lock couch at the correct height for the patient or ensure steps are available
2 members of staff assist the patient out of the chair —
  1 holding the chair
  1 supporting the patient
Care with urinary drainage bags and catheters, fractures, wounds
Sit patient on the couch
Allow time for patient to rest
Assist patient into position on the couch
Reverse the procedure when assisting the patient off the couch.

Lifting a patient from a wheelchair to the table

Place wheelchair near the table
2 people required to assist the patient
Explain procedure to the patient
Move the patient forward — until sitting on the edge of the chair
Stand either side of the patient facing the back of the chair
Place shoulder nearest patient under the patient's axilla
Place arm nearest patient under patient's thighs
Clasp the wrist of the other lifter, right hand grasps left wrist
Patient's arms hang over lifter's back
Support patient's back with free hand
Lifters bend knees and keeping their backs straight, lift the patient
Sit patient on table
Lift patient's legs onto the table.

PATIENTS IN BED

To raise to a sitting position

Explain procedure to the patient
2 people are required
Stand either side of the bed, facing the head of the bed
Place forearm of arm nearest the patient under patient's axilla
Bend knees, back straight
Carefully raise patient.

To move the patient up the bed

Explain the procedure to the patient

Raise the patient to the sitting position
Ask patient to bend his/her knees
Place forearm nearest the patient under the patient's axilla
Bend knees, back straight, lift the patient up the bed
At the same time patient pushes on the bed to assist (patient only asked to assist if able).

To lift the patient e.g. to place a cassette underneath

Explain procedure to the patient
3 people required, 2 to lift, 1 to position the cassette
Lifters stand at one side of the bed, feet apart and positioned in the direction of the movement, the third person is at the other side of the bed
Lifters bend knees, place arms under patient's shoulders and buttocks
Lift, keeping back straight, arms close to the body
Third person positions the cassette
Patient is gently lowered
To remove the cassette — reverse the procedure.

6. Inflammation and infection

INTRODUCTION

This section on inflammation and infection should be linked with the notes on hygiene, sterilisation and asepsis. In order to understand how infection can be controlled and the spread prevented it is necessary to have some basic knowledge of types of bacteria and the inflammatory process. There is no attempt to cover this vast subject in any detail because it is intended as an aid to help the student radiographer grasp the concept of what infection and sterilisation means in the confines of the clinical department.

INFLAMMATION

This is the reaction of vascular and supporting elements of tissues to various traumatic occurrences.
The inflammatory process should
> Limit the agent damaging the tissues
> Render the organisms harmless
> Repair the area of damage.

Causes

Invasion by micro-organisms e.g. bacteria
Mechanical trauma
Thermal trauma e.g. burns
Chemical trauma e.g. acids
Electrical trauma
Radiation trauma.

Local effects of inflammation

Pain and tenderness — due to tissue sensitivity ('stretching') and pressure on sensory nerve endings

Redness and heat — dilation of blood vessels

Swelling — increased blood supply and blood flow with alteration of blood vessel walls which changes osmo regulation, allowing fluid to flow into the tissue spaces

Loss of function

Formation of pus — formed by tissue and serum fluid, cellular constituents, living and dead bacteria.

Systemic effects (if the local reaction is not contained)

Pyrexia
Anorexia
Leucocytosis
Increased pulse and respiration rate
Decreased urinary output
Nausea/vomiting.

Cellular reaction to infection

Increase in polymorphonuclear leucocytes — particularly neutrophils which ingest bacteria by phagocytosis.

Monocytes ingest polymorphs and debris.

Lymphocytes produce antibodies against invading pathogens.

Pathogens produce a complex protein around themselves — an antigen. This triggers lymphocytes to manufacture specific antibodies against the antigen.

Antitoxin can be manufactured to neutralise toxins which may be produced by some pathogens e.g. tetanus produces a neurotoxin affecting the central nervous system.

Factors affecting healing

Poor diet
Poor blood supply to the area
Infection.

BACTERIA

Unicellular micro-organisms, most are harmless in their natural environment.

PATHOGENS

Bacteria causing disease
Examples:
Cocci — round in shape
Arranged in clusters — Staphylococcus aureus (Fig. 6.1)
Arranged in chains — Streptococcus (Fig. 6.2)
Arranged in pairs — Diplococcus pneumonius (Fig. 6.3).
Bacilli — rod shaped (Fig. 6.4)
Salmonella species
Clostridium perfringens
Spirochaete — thready spirals (Fig. 6.5)
Treponema pallidum
Most bacteria can be gram stained
    Positive — blue stain
    Negative — red stain

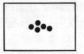

Fig. 6.1 Staphylococcus

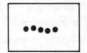

Fig. 6.2 Streptococcus

Fig. 6.3 Diplococcus

Fig. 6.4 Bacilli

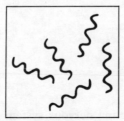

Fig. 6.5 Spirochaete

Characteristics of pathogens

Average size — 0.2–1.0 micron diameter, 0.5–4.0 micron length (spirochaete much longer)

Table 6.1 Gram stains

Organisms	Gram stain	Diseases produced
Staphylococcus aureus	Positive	Boils, wound infections
Streptococcus	Positive	Sore throats, tonsilitis
Diplococcus	Positive	Pneumonia
Salmonella	Negative	Food poisoning, Enteric fevers
Clostridium perfringens	Positive	Gas gangrene
Treponema pallidum	—	Syphilis

Motility — All cocci incapable of movement. Others possess flagella allowing whip-like movement.

Food requirements — Most bacteria need organic material.

Oxygen requirements — Most need oxygen — aerobic bacteria without oxygen — anaerobic bacteria.

Temperature requirements — Optimum temperature for most pathogens is 37°C.

Spore formation — Some bacteria are capable of producing a protective outer coating which protects the bacteria from heat and disinfectants e.g. tubercle bacillus and anthrax.

VIRUSES

Consist of:
A core of nucleic acid — DNA or RNA
Surrounded by a protein coat
Often enclosed in a lipid envelope
When invading a cell it takes complete control, using it for growth and reproduction.
Cell destruction follows.

Types of virus

Poliomyelitis   )
) affecting nervous system
Rabies   )

Smallpox)
)
Chickenpox) affecting skin
)
Measles)

Viral carcinogenesis

Some viruses are thought to have tumour inducing properties. Epstein-Barr virus (DNA virus) plus malaria is thought to produce Burkitt's lymphoma which is endemic in children in parts of Africa.

Fungal infections

Plant micro-organism usually multicellular e.g. Candida albicans (thrush).

Protozoa

Animal micro-organism e.g. amoeba, causes a type of dysentery.

INFECTION

A condition in which the body or part of the body is invaded by a pathogen which, under favourable conditions multiplies and produces injurious effects.

Localised infection is usually accompanied by inflammation.

Endogenous infection

Derived from host person
Harmful only when transferred to a non-acceptable site e.g. pathogen Escherichia coli from bowel can produce a urinary tract infection.

Exogenous infection

Infection transmitted from one person to another — either from a carrier (often with undiagnosed infections) or from a person with a diagnosed infection.

Spread of infection

By direct contact
During a surgical operation, therefore anything touching the patient should be sterile.

By indirect contact
   Through water — typhoid, cholera
   Through animals — rabies
   Through insects — malaria
   Through the air — droplets transmitting influenza, dust and fluff
Once the organism has gained entry into the body it may spread by various routes:
   Through tissue spaces — cellulitis
   Through the lymphatic vessels — lymphadenitis
   Through the circulatory system — septicaemia
   Passages between two anatomically separate organs — fistula formation
   Capillary deposits — abscesses (bacteria in capillaries — pyaemia), may form abnormal channels to skin surfaces called sinuses.

CROSS INFECTION

Occurs when an infection is transferred from one person to another
General measures to control the spread of infection include
   High standards in personal, departmental and equipment hygiene (see Hygiene section)

When dealing with a patient with an infection ensure that

   Treatment room/imaging room, equipment and changing cubicles are damp dusted with disinfectant impregnated cloths
   Correct disposal of infected articles is carried out
   Disposable linen is used at all times
   Accessory equipment is covered
   There is correctly functioning air conditioning
   Appointment for patient given at the end of the working day or when the department is not busy
   Local infection control policies will apply via the Infection Control Manager.

NOTIFIABLE DISEASES

In October 1988, the Acheson Report on Public Health Regulations passed into law.

Notifiable diseases are a group of diseases which must be notified to the Medical Officer for Environmental Health by the diagnosing medical officer/pathologist.

Accurate notification aids:

Effective control of disease and preventative measures

Assessment of medical policies, service provision and immunisation programmes

Statutory notifiable diseases in England and Wales include: mumps, rubella, poliomyelitis, smallpox, venereal disease, tuberculosis, infectious hepatitis (this is not a complete list).

AIDS is not a notifiable disease.

The reporting system should be computerised and link with Local Health Authority, Public Health Laboratory service and General Practitioner practices.

ISOLATION TECHNIQUES

Source isolation

For patients with serious contagious diseases, isolation of pathogen may be required.

General measures

Single room

Warning notice outside room

Plastic apron and gloves when handling patient or body fluids

Minimal traffic to and from room

Special procedures for linen removal and disposable items

Special instructions for cleaning staff.

Strict isolation — required for patients with diseases such as meningitis, anthrax

Use of plastic gowns and gloves

Masks should be worn

Staff should be immunised where appropriate.

Radiography

Two radiographers required

First radiographer positions the patient and cassette
Second radiographer uses the equipment
Radiographers should wear plastic apron and gloves, and masks
Cassette placed in a disposable waterproof cover.

After the exposure

First radiographer removes the cassette, holding the cover
Second radiographer removes the cassette from the cover.

After the examination

Wash hands, remove protective clothing, wash hands again.

Protective isolation

For patients with incompetent immune system
Severe burns
Transplant recipients
Patients receiving high dose total body irradiation.

General measures

Single room
No plants or flowers
Specific cleaning procedures e.g. damp dusting
Nursing staff should be free from infections
Careful handwashing with antiseptic solution e.g. triclosan
Plastic aprons and masks are worn by staff
Special air conditioning with filtered air
Equipment such as thermometers, stethoscopes etc. sterilised prior
to use and not removed from room
Visiting of patient carefully monitored, masks worn, hands washed.

Laminar flow isolation

Unit can be placed on main ward
Large plastic tent
Filtered air pumped in
Anti-infection precautions, as above
Reduces problems of isolation.

TOTAL BODY IRRADIATION (TBI)

Prior to bone marrow transplants

Care of the patient

Following TBI, patients develop acute leucopenia
Protective isolation techniques are required
Prophylactic antibiotic cover
Hickman line inserted prior to treatment — strict aseptic techniques
Patient has pre-sterilised food, avoiding yoghurt, ice creams, salad
Sterilised fluids only
Fluid balance recordings
Temperature, pulse, respiration and blood pressure recorded 4 hourly.

INFECTION IN PATIENTS WITH MALIGNANT DISEASE

Infections in patients with malignant disease are a major cause of death.
    These patients are more susceptible to infection — depression of host defence mechanisms by tumour and its treatment.

Localised infection

Infection in tumour area reduces the effectiveness of radiotherapy
Blood supply may be impaired, oxygen tension reduced
Anoxic cells are resistant to photon radiation
Impaired blood supply delays healing processes
Irradiation of carious teeth accelerates dental decay
Dental extractions should be performed prior to treatment
Patients are at risk of contracting systemic and opportunistic infections if:

total leucocyte count less than	4.0×10^9/litre
lymphocytes less than	1.5×10^9/litre
neutrophils less than	1.5×10^9/litre

ACQUIRED IMMUNE DEFICIENCY SYNDROME (AIDS)

AIDS is a contagious viral disease.
The virus (HIV) attacks the immune system of the body.

Patients who have infected blood which is HIV antibody positive fall into one of four categories:

Symptom free carriers
Have no outward sign of the infection.

Persistent generalised lymphadenopathy (PGL)
Have swollen glands but feel well.

AIDS related complex (ARC)
Complain of being tired, night sweats and weight loss
Suffer from infections

Acquired immune deficiency syndrome (AIDS)
(About 10% of infected patients)
Are ill and have life-threatening disease(s) e.g. Kaposi sarcoma, pneumocystis pneumonia.

NB. An infected person who at the time of blood testing has not produced antibodies can still pass on the infection.

Transmission of the AIDS virus

AIDS is a sexually transmitted disease, transmitted principally by sexual intercourse
Condoms reduce the risk of infection
AIDS can be caught from infected blood:
On a shared needle
Via a blood transfusion (all blood and blood products are screened and treated in the UK).
By children born to mothers who are HIV positive.

Professional responsibilities

Patient confidentiality must be respected
All patients must be treated with sensitivity and respect
It is unprofessional to refuse to work with an infected patient
All blood and body fluids from ALL patients must be treated as potentially hazardous.

Precautions for staff

Broken skin must be covered with waterproof dressings
Staff who have an accident involving blood or body fluids are advised to have their serum tested
Needles should be disposed of, unsheathed, in a sharps box

Gloves should be worn when there is a risk of coming into contact with body fluids

Local control of infection protocol should be read and followed.

Accidental exposure to AIDS virus and other high risk infections

If you come into contact with patient's body fluids:
Unbroken skin — wash with soap and running water, do not scrub
Broken skin — wash with soap and running water; remove waterproof dressing; wash with soap and running water, do not scrub
Splashes, mouth or eyes — rinse with running water
If injury occurs — encourage wound to bleed; wash with soap and water, do not scrub
Report incident to the head of department
Fill in an accident form
Notify occupational health staff.

Collection of specimens from high risk patients

Clearly labelled with Bio-Hazard Warning label
Must be handled by the minimum number of people
Should be taken to pathology department
Should be handed to a member of staff
Should not be left in reception areas.

Suggested departmental protocol for patients who are suffering from infection, haemorrhage, incontinent, vomiting, have open skin lesions, unconscious, mentally disturbed or confused

Imaging should be done with mobile equipment
Wear: gown, plastic apron, plastic gloves
Additional protective clothing: where splashing may occur
Cassette and accessories: waterproof cover
Disposal of clothing and waste: double bagged in plastic sacks, sealed with tape, labelled with hazard warning and incinerated
Spillage: cover with 2% glutaraldehyde, leave for 1 minute, mop up with paper towels, wipe with same solution
Contamination of wounds: wash with soap and hot water

Resuscitation equipment: direct mouth to mouth resuscitation should not be used, equipment e.g. Brook airway, should be available
Use and care of mobile imaging equipment: after leaving the room the radiographer
    Removes, gown, apron and gloves
    Puts on new gown, apron and gloves
    Isolates the equipment from the mains
    Wipes the machine with 70% ethyl or isopropyl alcohol
    Removes gown, apron and gloves
    Correctly disposes of all protective clothing.

Other imaging and radiotherapy techniques

Patient should be at the end of the list
All non-essential equipment should be removed from the area
Couch/table covered with water-repellant laminate
Staff follow infection protocol
After the examination
Isolate the equipment from the mains
Clean with 70% ethyl or isopropyl alcohol
For further information see Control of Infection Protocol (College of Radiographers 1990).

DISPOSAL OF WASTE

All hospital waste disposal should be covered by a policy approved by the Department of Health (DOH) and the Health and Safety Commission.

Examples

Household waste — paper articles
Stored in container on bin
Sealed daily
Incinerated
Clinical waste containing body fluids/tissue
Placed in colour coded bag, sealed, labelled
Minimum storage time
Incinerated.
Sharps
(Needles, scalpels, broken ampoules, cannulae)

Disposal of sharps is responsibility of user
40% of needle stick injuries occur at attempted resheathing
Use of DOH approved sharps box
  Place on even surface with good visibility
  Do not resheath needles
  Close box when two thirds full
  Do not separate needle from syringe manually
  Glass which may be too large for sharps box — disposed of in a
  labelled rigid container (assuming no biohazard)

7. Sterilisation

INTRODUCTION

This chapter deals with the sterilisation procedures which are available for various articles used daily by radiographers.

It is important that inadequately sterilised articles are recognised and discarded, therefore a knowledge of the principles involved in these procedures is necessary.

Student radiographers should be shown how to store sterilised articles and packs and to use stock in the correct order.

Sterilisation is the complete removal of living organisms from an object or body.

Methods available

Moist heat — Autoclaving
                Boiling (emergency only)
Dry heat — Hot air oven
             Infra-red oven
Chemical — Liquid–immersion
              Gases–autoclave
Gamma radiation.

MOIST HEAT — AUTOCLAVING

The autoclave (Fig. 7.1)

Has 2 shells — the outer called the jacket
               the inner called the chamber
A hinged access door
Articles are packed loosely in an inner chamber
Chamber is evacuated by a vacuum pump
Steam under pressure is introduced into the jacket and chamber

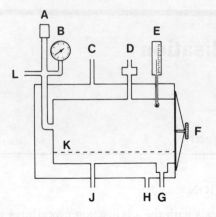

Fig. 7.1 Diagram showing a section through an autoclave
A — Safety valve
B — Pressure gauge
C — Steam inlet to jacket
D — Air inlet to chamber
E — Temperature gauge
F — Safety door
G — Chamber exhaust
H — Jacket exhaust
J — Steam extractor
K — Trivet
L — Steam inlet

The steam is at a set temperature and pressure and is introduced
for a set time
Steam is removed
Articles are dried in situ
Filtered air is reintroduced.

Tests for efficiency

Barograph recording

Pressure, temperature and holding time recorded for each run.

Bowie and Dick Test (daily)

36 huckaback towels are folded to make a pile 270 mm high and
are packed in a sealed container
2 pieces of autoclave tape are placed between them (autoclave

tape has equal brown stripes if sterile, no stripes if not)
Autoclave is run
If all the tape has brown stripes and the towels are dry the autoclave
is working.

Brown's tubes

Glass phial containing a fluid which changes colour if the autoclave
is working correctly
Used for each run.

Articles for autoclaving

Articles must be socially clean and are either washed mechanically
or cleaned with ultrasound
Double wrapped paper packets must allow steam to enter
Articles must be dry
Linen must be clean and laundered, then packed in paper
Autoclave tape is used to secure the paper or the packets have a
heat sensitive panel.

Articles suitable

Instruments (non-disposable)
Linen
Dressings

Articles unsuitable

Plastic items
Most disposable items.

Typical programme

250 kilopascals (kPa) at 135°C for 3–3.5 minutes
Articles are allowed to cool and dry.

After autoclaving

Check — Tape is striped
          Seal is not broken
          Packs are dry.

MOIST HEAT — BOILING (emergency use only)

Disadvantages

No standardisation
Time consuming
Easily contaminated
No check on the sterility of the articles
Spores are not destroyed and as some bacteria are spore forming
there is a risk of infection.

DRY HEAT

Hot air oven

Articles are either washed mechanically or by ultrasound
Packaged in metal containers, glass tubes or are double wrapped
with aluminium foil
An indicator is placed on the package
Socially clean articles placed in the oven
Articles must not be tightly packed
Articles are allowed to cool before removal.

Typical programme

170°C for 1 hour.

Articles suitable

Hardened delicate glasswear
Delicate instruments and needles
All glass syringes.

Articles unsuitable

Rubber
Plastic

GAMMA RADIATION

Unit

Socially clean articles placed on a moving conveyor belt
Radiation source is of short wavelength.

Typical dosage

2.5×10^4 Gray (Gy).

Sterile packs

Have a red dot if sterile
Or are marked gamma ray sterilised.

Articles suitable

Those which would be damaged by heat
Plastic catheters
Knife holders
Disposable instruments, gloves etc.

CHEMICAL

Principles

Articles — must be socially clean
must be submerged for the required length of time
Chemical — either in solution or gaseous
must be sufficiently strong
more effective hot than cold
Container — must be sterile
can be an autoclave.

Types of chemical

Bacteriocidal — agent kills bacteria
Bacteriostatic — agent inhibits growth of bacteria
Antiseptic — inhibits growth of bacteria.

Chemical gas

Ethylene oxide — used in an autoclave at 55°C and 220 kilopascals
for 3 hours
Suitable for most plastics
Has a yellow dot if sterile.

Liquid disinfectants

Alcohol — skin preparation
Cetrimide — skin disinfection
Chlorhexidine — skin disinfection
Chlorinated solutions — wound cleaning
Iodine compounds — skin disinfection.

CENTRAL STERILE SUPPLY DEPARTMENT (CSSD)

Supplies departments with prepacked sterile items

Advantages

Standardisation of pack contents
Packs available at short notice
Labour saving
Less handling of articles
Packs are available for specific procedures.

Disadvantages

Transportation between the unit and department may be difficult
Over ordering could result in wastage

Presentation

Packs double wrapped with water repellent paper
Drums and boxes are used

Use of CSSD packs

A record book is used when ordering packs
Store packs in a cool, dry, well ventilated place
Packs used in strict rotation.
Check
  Correct pack
  Expiry date/date of sterilisation
  Either an indicator panel or autoclave tape shows if the pack is
  sterile
  Tape is striped

    Seal is not broken
    Pack is dry
Open outer pack
Shake the contents onto a sterile surface
Open contents, touching the outside cover only
After use, clean and return articles.

8. Instruments and dressings

INTRODUCTION

This section is intended as an introduction to some of the instruments and dressings which the student radiographer may come across during the training period.

Although radiographers will not have direct responsibility for the use of some of the instruments, it is desirable for them to understand how the instruments are used.

It is usual for students to be taught about instruments and dressings under clinical supervision, which should enable the students to develop a competent practical technique when called upon to assist in any procedures involving the use of instruments and dressings.

Biopsy forceps (Fig. 8.1)

Long metal forceps with crocodile action of the end blades, used for taking tissue samples from narrow passages e.g. the throat. They operate with a scissor action. Must be sterilised before use.

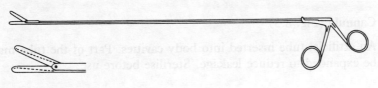

Fig. 8.1 Biopsy forceps

Brook airway (Fig. 8.2)

Used for expired air ventilation to avoid direct contact with the patient. The mouth guard provides a seal over the patient's mouth.

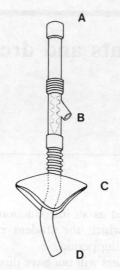

Fig. 8.2 Brook airway
A — Operator's mouth piece
B — Exit port for patient's exhaled air
C — Mouth guard
D — Patient's mouth piece

Patient's exhaled air escapes through an exhaust port. Socially clean before use.

Catheters (excluding urinary catheters)

Tubing of either rubber or plastic for the introduction of substances into the body. Sterilise before use.

Cannula (Fig. 8.3)

An artificial tube inserted into body cavities. Part of the tube may be expanded to reduce leakage. Sterilise before use.

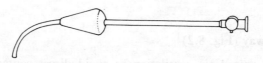

Fig. 8.3 Cannula

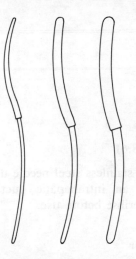

Fig. 8.4 Cervical dilators

Cervical dilator (Fig. 8.4)

Metal instrument used to dilate the cervix e.g. prior to the insertion of radioactive caesium uterine applicators or prior to hysterosalpingography. Sterilise before use.

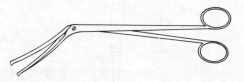

Fig. 8.5 Cheatle forceps

Cheatle forceps (Fig. 8.5)
Long handled forceps
Kept in a jar of disinfectant
2 pairs required
Always hold with points down to prevent contamination of the forceps
Do not allow them to touch nonsterile objects

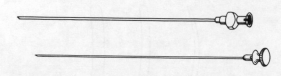

Fig. 8.6 Chiba needle

Chiba needle (Fig. 8.6)

A 15 cm long, thin, stainless steel needle used to inject a contrast agent directly into an intrahepatic duct during percutaneous cholangiography. Sterilise before use.

Clinical thermometer

Used for taking the patient's temperature, may be of oral, rectal or low temperature type. Sterilise before use.

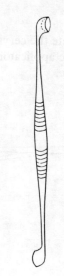

Fig. 8.7 Curette

Curette (Fig. 8.7)

A double, spoon ended, instrument for reducing or excising a basal cell carcinoma. Sterilise before use.

Drip infusion sets

Consist of a bottle, tubing and a needle. Used for introducing a substance into a patient over a long period of time, e.g. infusion cholangiography, chemotherapy drugs. Sterile procedure — apart from rectal infusion.

Endotracheal tube

Passed down the trachea to maintain a clear airway, used in anaesthetics and may be cuffed or uncuffed. Sterilise before use.

Forceps

Cheatle forceps. Long handled forceps, usually metal, used for removing sterile instruments out of solution. Must always be held with the points down. Sterilise before use.

Dissecting forceps (Fig. 8.8). Used for picking up 'light' articles (heavy articles turn the blades out of true). Used during biopsies and for performing sterile dressings using no-touch technique. Sterilise before use.

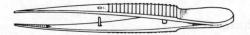

Fig. 8.8 Dissecting forceps — non toothed

Sponge holding forceps (Fig. 8.9). Rounded ends, used for holding swabs when cleaning a patient e.g. prior to femoral arteriography or hysterosalpingography. Sterilise before use.

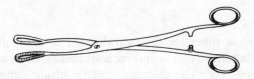

Fig. 8.9 Sponge holding forceps

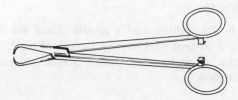

Fig. 8.10 Tissue forceps

Tissue forceps (Fig. 8.10). Pointed ends which can be clipped together, used for holding the skin. Sterilise before use.

Gallipots

Either plastic or tin foil (disposable) or metal (reusable) bowls used to hold solutions. Sterilise before use.

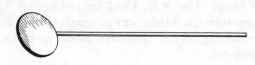

Fig. 8.11 Laryngeal mirror

Laryngeal mirror (Fig. 8.11)

Small mirror on a metal rod, used for examining the oral cavity and during indirect laryngoscopies. Socially clean before use.

Laryngoscope

An instrument used to inspect the larynx visually during direct laryngoscopy to see if there is any obstruction present, and can be used to take tissue samples if necessary. Sterilise before use.

Needles

Pointed narrow tubes for the introduction of substances, by subcutaneous, intramuscular or intravenous means, or to aspirate fluid. Usually disposable. The coloured, plastic fitting denotes the size. Sterilise before use.

Lumbar puncture needle. Long needle used for performing a lumbar puncture, for the removal of cerebrospinal fluid or the introduction of a contrast agent or chemotherapy drugs. Sterilise before use.

Drawing up needle. Long, wide ended needle used for filling syringes. Sterilise before use.

Sialography needle. Used for injecting contrast agents into the salivary glands. Metal, with an expanded area to prevent the agent from spilling out of the gland. Sterilise before use.

Ophthalmoscope

Instrument for examining the eye. Consists of a mirror with a hole in it, through which the observer looks. The inner aspect of the eye (retina) is illuminated by light reflected from the mirror. Can be fitted with different size lenses. Socially clean before use.

Pneumatic cuff

Rubber/fabric cuff, wrapped round the arm/leg and expanded with air. Used to occlude an artery or measure the blood pressure. Maximum time for which it should be inflated on the patient's limb is 10 minutes or gangrene may result. Socially clean before use.

Proctoscope

Endoscope with a light source used to inspect the rectum visually. Socially clean before use.

Receiver

Large metal bowl used to receive dirty swabs and instruments usually during a sterile procedure. Socially clean before use.

Seldinger trocar and cannula (Fig. 8.12)

Used for the introduction of a guide wire/catheter into an artery. The trocar has a pointed end, and fits inside the cannula (more than one trocar may be required if a large cannula is used). Both are introduced, the trocar is removed and the guide wire is inserted through the cannula. The catheter is then fed over the guide wire.

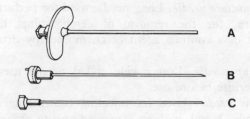

Fig. 8.12 Seldinger trocar and cannula
A — Cannula
B — Trocar
C — Stilette

Can be used to insert a cannula to drain fluid from a cavity. Sterilise before use.

Scalpel blades

Usually disposable metal blade (and plastic holder) used in surgery for opening the skin surface. Sterilise before use.

Sphygmomanometer

Instrument for measuring the blood pressure. Socially clean before use.

Surgical masks

Cloth/paper and polythene/paper masks which cover the nose and mouth. Paper masks worn for a maximum of 10 minutes, must be changed if become moist.

Swabs

Pieces of gauze or paper material for cleaning, packing superficial wounds. Sterilise before use.

Filamented swabs — have a radiopaque strip. Used in theatre for internal swabbing as the swab can be traced radiographically if lost. Sterilise before use.

Syringes

Either plastic (disposable) or glass and metal (reusable) have graduated markings on the side and an end fitting. Sterilise before use.

Higginson's syringe — rubber syringe with a balloon and a one way valve. Used for pumping air e.g. into the rectum during a barium enema. Socially clean before use.

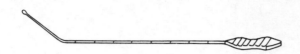

Fig. 8.13 Uterine sound

Uterine sound (Fig. 8.13)

Long, blunt ended, curved instrument with a scale on the side. Used for assessing the length and direction of the uterus prior to hysterosalpingography. Sterilise before use.

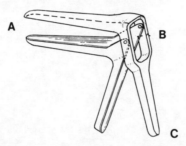

Fig. 8.14 Vaginal speculum
A — Inserted into the vagina
B — For the introduction of instruments
C — Handles

Vaginal speculum (Fig. 8.14)

Metal or plastic instrument inserted into the vagina to enable the examination of the cervix and uterus and to allow the introduction of instruments. Sterilise before use.

Victoria enema ring

Circular, rubber disc, the rim of which can be inflated with air, used during barium enema examinations to contain the barium in the event of involuntary defaecation. Socially clean before use.

Vomit bowls

Metal/plastic/paper bowls with a long handle used to receive vomit. Socially clean before use.

9. Patient preparation — diagnostic

INTRODUCTION

Every patient who enters an imaging department will require some form of preparation. It is important that the student radiographer understands that such routine checks such as the patient's full name and address must be carried out carefully or a situation may occur which leads to the wrong patient being radiographed.

The importance of correct abdominal preparation cannot be over-emphasised as faecal matter may obscure small detail in the abdomen such as renal calculi. All staff are advised to check, at regular intervals, the current patient preparation in use in the department.

A chart at the end of the chapter outlines the patient preparation before and after specific examinations. The preparation may vary from department to department because of individual preference and therefore example preparations only are given.

Preparation may take place immediately prior to a radiographic examination or may extend over several days.

EXPOSURE OF IONISING RADIATION TO WOMEN WHO ARE OR MAY BE PREGNANT

When radiographing a female patient of childbearing age, where the uterus is in or near the useful beam, the radiographer is responsible for establishing that the patient is not pregnant.

It is important that the radiographer is familiar with the checking procedure which should be displayed in the department.

The patient should be asked, in private, the pregnancy question, which is: 'Are you, or might you be pregnant?' If any answer but no is given, ask the date of the last menstrual period and record the answer.

Consult the referring clinician/radiologist. Record that the procedure has been followed.

OUT PATIENT PREPARATION

The patient should be given written details of:
  Time and date of the examination
  A simple explanation of the examination
  Full details of any preparation required
  Approximate length of time of the examination
  Name of the hospital and department
  Hospital telephone number and department extension
NB. The possibility of pregnancy should be considered when booking an appointment for female patients of childbearing age when the uterus is in or near the useful beam.

IN PATIENT PREPARATION

The information should be sent to the Ward Sister/Charge nurse of the ward concerned.
  Name and record number of the patient
  Date and time of the examination
  Nature of the examination
  Details of any preparation required

GENERAL PREPARATION

Ask the patient his/her name and check with the request form
Check the patient's:
  Address
  Age
  Occupation
  Ward (if applicable)
Ask the pregnancy question (if applicable)
Ask if the patient has been radiographed before, if so where and when
Ask if they have followed any instructions which may have been given previously
Check if any adverse effects have occurred following the ingestion of any tablets/medicines, or earlier X-ray examinations
Give a full explanation of any clothing which has to be removed
Ensure clean gown and dressing gown are available.

PREPARATION FOR ABDOMINAL EXAMINATIONS

It is necessary to remove intestinal gas and faeces which may obscure visualisation of small detail e.g. renal calculi, gall stones.

FLATULENCE

This is the presence of excessive gas in the gastro-intestinal tract.

Causes

Nervous stress — Causing muscle spasm. Air swallowing (aerophagy)
Diet — High carbohydrate intake. High fat intake
Immobility — Patient may be bedridden
Patient may have a limited range of movement
Preparation — The over-use of aperients
Inadequate explanation/reassurance
Drugs/drinks — Carbonated drinks.

Prevention

Reassurance — Prevents the patient from worrying
Recommend no smoking, to prevent aerophagy (NB. this may cause gas if the patient becomes anxious without cigarettes)
Low roughage diet (low residue) — e.g. mince, mashed vegetables, fish, milk based foods
Activity — Encourage movement/exercise
Aperients — Ensure the recommended dose is not exceeded
(Note list of contraindications under aperients)

Elimination

Drugs

  e.g. Hyoscine butylbromide 2, 10 mg tablets

Charcoal tablets or biscuits
  Prescribed because charcoal absorbs gas

Flatus tube

  Thick rectal tube with an expanded end opening
  Tube connected to a funnel

Rounded end of tube lubricated and inserted into the rectum
Funnel placed under water so that the gas can be seen escaping

FAECES

Waste products of digestion

Elimination

Diet. A laxative effect can be obtained by a diet that contains
sufficient roughage e.g. fruits, vegetables

Aperients — Induce gentle peristaltic action of the bowel causing
defaecation. NB. Large doses can cause pain, spasm, diarrhoea,
flatulence.

Faecal softeners — These lubricate the colon wall and ease the
passage of softened faecal matter e.g. liquid paraffin.

Bulk producing — The contents retain water and mix with the
intestinal contents to form a soft mass which encourages peristalsis. May take several days to develop e.g. bran.

Stimulant laxatives — Stimulate colonic peristalsis e.g. sodium
picosulphate with magnesium citrate, Picolax — 10 mg in water in
the morning and the afternoon of the day prior to the examination.
Used in conjunction with a low residue diet with plenty of water;
bisacodyl — 2 × 5 mg at night 2 days prior, if necessary 10 mg
suppository 1 hour prior.

Contraindications for the use of aperients

Haemorrhage/obstruction of the alimentary tract
Ulcerative colitis
Diverticulosis/diverticulitis
Diarrhoea
Megacolon
Young children

Enematic and colonic lavage

Enema

Fluid is introduced into the colon per rectum, or via a colostomy
To remove faecal matter from the bowel
To replace lost body fluids
To administer drugs

To remove faecal matter

Fluids used:
  Phosphate enemas
Trolley setting:
  Lubricant on a swab
  Disposable towel
  Container for the solution
  Catheter/tubing
  Clips
  Bedpan/commode
Procedure:
  Explanation and reassurance
  Screens placed round the patient
  Patient lies on their left side, hips and knees flexed
  Protective sheet is placed under the patient
  Air is expelled from the funnel and catheter by running through some liquid and clamping off the tubing
  Catheter is lubricated and inserted into the rectum
  Approximately 1 litre of solution is administered, at a temperature of 5°C
  Catheter is removed
  Patient is asked to retain the enema for 3 minutes
  Patient is placed on a bedpan and the bowel contents are evacuated
  Patient is cleaned and made comfortable.

Colonic lavage

Performed to empty the bowel prior to examination or operation.
Fluid used:
  Water
Trolley setting:
  See Enema
Procedure:
  Patient lies on their left side, hips and knees flexed
  Catheter inserted into the rectum
  Solution is administered
  Solution is 'run out' through the catheter
  Process continues until clear fluid returns.

Diet modification

Patient may be requested to have nothing to eat or drink prior to the examination e.g. if a general anaesthetic is required or in opaque meals (e.g. barium).

Patient follows a low roughage diet for 48 hours prior e.g. Minced meat, fish etc. avoiding green vegetables, cereals, whole meal bread, fatty foods.

Patient avoids gas forming foods e.g. parsnips, peas, beans, effervescent drinks and starchy foods.

Patients who require special care

Diabetic patients

Medical consultation prior to diet modification
Given laxatives only
Always placed first on a list
If the patient has to starve, told to omit insulin and bring food and insulin with him.

Children

No abdominal preparation required.

Bed patients

Encouraged to sit up or if possible walk around to avoid flatulence.

Example of a typical abdominal preparation

Low roughage diet 48 hours prior
Avoid gas forming foods 48 hours prior
Laxative given 36 and 12 hours prior to the examination.

NURSING CARE BEFORE AND AFTER SPECIFIC EXAMINATIONS

Before all examinations it is essential that
    The patient's identity is checked
    They are given a full explanation of the procedure
    They are reassured
    The patient is asked the pregnancy question, if appropriate
    Emergency drugs are available when iodine-based contrast agents are used
After all examinations the patient is told:
    When they can return to a normal diet
    When and where they can get the results

Examination	Definition	Patient preparation before the examination	Patient care after the examination
Angiography (general)	Demonstration of the circulatory system by the injection of an iodine based contrast agent into an artery	Abdominal preparation may be required Consent form signed Premedication given Nothing by mouth 5 hours prior Warned of metallic taste following injection of the contrast agent	Observe injection site for haematoma following digital pressure Spray injection site with plastic skin dressing Pulse and blood pressure taken every 30 minutes for 4 hours Then every 4 hours for 24 hours
Carotid angiography	Demonstration of the brain circulation by direct injection into the carotid artery or via a catheter in the femoral artery, which is passed to the carotid artery	See angiography (general) Shave groin if femoral catheter used	See angiography (general)
Femoral arteriography	Catheter inserted into a palpable artery in the leg (usually femoral)	See angiography (general)	See angiography (general)

Examination	Definition	Patient preparation before the examination	Patient care after the examination
Translumbar aortography	Investigation of the aorta and major branches by direct injection into the abdominal aorta	See angiography (general) Shave as necessary	See angiography (general)
Arch aortography	Investigation of the aorta and major branches by femoral or axillary catheterisation	See angiography (general) Shave as necessary (groin or axilla)	See angiography (general)
Renal arteriography	Investigation of the renal areas by catheterisation of the femoral artery	See angiography (general) Micturate prior to the examination Shave groin	See angiography (general)
Angiocardio-graphy (cardiac catheterisation)	Demonstration of the heart and great vessels by brachial or femoral catheterisation	See angiography (general) Shave as necessary	See angiography (general)
Arthrography (e.g. knee)	Investigation of joint anatomy following the injection of air or a low osmolarity contrast agent into the joint capsule	Preliminary films taken Knee shaved Transport home arranged	Rest with limb elevated for 12 hours
Opaque meal e.g. barium	Examination of the stomach by the ingestion of a radiopaque contrast agent	Abdominal preparation Nothing by mouth 8 hours prior Warn of possible follow through examination	Ensure mouth is clean Warn of possible constipation Inform the patient that he can return to normal diet

Opaque swallow e.g. barium	Examination of the oesophagus by the ingestion of a radiopaque contrast agent	As for a barium meal	As for a barium meal
Opaque enema e.g. barium	Examination of the colon by the introduction of a radiopaque contrast agent or a radiopaque and radiolucent contrast agent, via rectal catheter or a colostomy	Sigmoidoscopy or colonoscopy performed to check the colon Abdominal preparation Asked to retain the contrast agent Informed of the evacuation stage Ensure toilet facilities are available	Warn of possible constipation Ensure clean and comfortable Provide a fresh bag for colostomy patients
Bronchography	Investigation of the bronchial tree following the introduction of contrast agent via the trachea	Postural drainage for 3 days prior Requested not to cough during the procedure Nothing by mouth for 5 hours prior Light premedication given Local anaesthetic may be required	Allowed to cough Nothing by mouth for 3 hours — warn of the danger of inhaling food or drink Postural drainage may be required
Oral cholecystography	Investigation of the biliary tract by the ingestion of a contrast agent	Preliminary film taken Abdominal preparation Fat free diet 12 hours prior Contrast agent taken in the evening prior to the examination and the morning of the examination Then nothing by mouth except fat free fluids	Return to normal diet

Examination	Definition	Patient preparation before the examination	Patient care after the examination
Endoscopic retrograde choledocho-pancreatography (ERCP)	Investigation of the pancreatic and biliary systems. The contrast agent is injected into the papilla of Vater via a fibre-optic endoscope	Nothing by mouth for 5 hours prior. Premedication given. Recent radiographs of the biliary tract area should be available. Pharynx is anaesthetised. Endoscope is introduced	Nothing by mouth for 2 hours. Serum amylase level is checked the following day (any rise in the level is indicative of pancreatitis)
Infusion cholangiography	Investigation of the biliary tract by infusion of a radiopaque contrast agent (undertaken when oral cholecystography has failed)	As for oral cholecystography but contrast agent given on the day of the examination. Checked for history of allergy. Arm prepared for an intravenous injection	Return to normal diet
Dacryocystography	Investigation of the lacrimal system following the direct injection of a radiopaque contrast agent	Local anaesthetic required	Eye covered until the 'blinking' action returns
Excretion urography	Investigation of the kidneys, ureters and bladder following injection of a radiopaque contrast agent	Abdominal preparation. Check for history of allergies. Patient asked to micturate prior to examination	Non-specific
Lymphography	Investigation of the lymphatic system following a direct injection of the contrast agent into a lymphatic vessel of the foot	If oedema of the leg, admitted for several days. Chest X-ray. Abdominal preparation. Dorsum of foot shaved	Pressure bandages applied to foot. Inform the patient that further films may be required. Keep foot dry because of sutures in situ

	Warn patient and relatives of change in skin colour Warn patient of change in urine colour and vision will have blue/green haze Empty bladder prior to examination	
Radiculography	Investigation of the spinal canal following the injection of water soluble contrast agent via a lumbar puncture	Recent radiographic examination of the spine Nothing by mouth for 5 hours prior to examination The contrast agent may be introduced on the ward	Pulse and blood pressure every 30 minutes for 4 hours Sudden movement should be avoided Trunk and head raised for 8 hours Bed rest for 24 hours
Retrograde pyelograph	Performed when an IU has failed Introduction of a catheter into the renal pelvis via the urethra and bladder to introduce a radiopaque contrast agent	Abdominal preparation Consent form signed Warned not to remove the catheter Starvation for 4 hours prior Premedication given General anaesthetic	4 hourly observations of temperature, pulse and respiration for 24 hours Return to normal diet
Cystography	The introduction of a radiopaque contrast agent into the bladder via a catheter	Empty bladder Requested to retain the contrast agent Toilet facilities available Nervous patients may require a sedative	May be given sulphonamides for 4 days following to counteract infection

Examination	Definition	Patient preparation before the examination	Patient care after the examination
Male urethro-graphy	Investigation of the male urethra following the introduction of a radiopaque contrast agent	Full explanation given Micturate prior to the examination Local anaesthetic given	Warned that haematuria may occur Sulphonamides may be prescribed
Hysterosalping-ography	Investigation of the uterus and uterine tubes following cannulation of the cervix	Examination takes place after menstruation and within the first 12 days of the menstrual cycle Empty bladder prior to the examination Premedication/general anaesthetic may be required Recovery room prepared	Patient rests if necessary Warned of possible haemorrhage Tampon/towel provided
Sialography	Investigation of the salivary glands following the direct injection of a radiopaque contrast agent	Preliminary films required Patient removes false teeth Patient is given a lemon to suck to open the ampulla of the duct	Mouthwash is given
Peripheral venography	Investigation of the venous system of a limb following direct injection of a radiopaque contrast agent into a vein	Nothing by mouth for 5 hours prior to the examination Micturate prior to the examination Premedication given	When premedication has worn off, encourage to walk about
Portal venography	Investigation of the portal system following the direct injection of a radiopaque contrast agent into the spleen	Abdominal preparation Micturate prior to examination Premedication given Nothing by mouth for 5 hours prior	Bed rest for 5 hours Pulse and blood pressure every 15 minutes for 4 hours Temperature, pulse, respiration, blood pressure every 4 hours for 24 hours Analgesics may be required

PATIENT PREPARATION FOR OTHER IMAGING TECHNIQUES

ULTRASOUND

General preparation

Check identity of the patient
Give explanation and reassurance
Removal of clothing from the area of interest
Ultrasonic gel spread over the area to be examined
Change the sheets between patients.

Preparation for specific examinations

Abdomen

Problem of bowel gas as this reflects ultrasonic waves
Abdominal preparation may be required
Practise breathing techniques
Should be no barium sulphate present in the patient as this prevents the passage of ultrasonic waves
Nothing by mouth for 5 hours prior — to ensure gall bladder is full of bile
If performed during cholecystography — should be prior to the fatty meal.

Obstetrics and gynaecology

Transabdominal

Full urinary bladder required — displaces bowel gas in early pregnancy and gives a 'window' to view the uterus and lifts the fetal head out of the pelvis in later pregnancy
Liaison with the antenatal clinic as patients are often requested to give a urine sample — ultrasound should be done first
Clinical history should be available
Patient may feel faint due to pressure of the fetus on the inferior vena cava. If this occurs turn the patient onto the side to relieve the pressure.

Transvaginal

All male staff must be chaperoned
Patient must be given the choice of techniques

Careful explanation is required
The patient must be assured of privacy
Strict rules of hygiene must be observed
The vaginal probe must not be used if the patient has no previous
sexual activity or if there is heavy vaginal bleeding.

Biopsy and aspiration techniques

Signed consent form required
Previous radiographs and case notes required
Aseptic technique
Patient should rest following the examination.

RADIONUCLIDE IMAGING

General preparation

Check the identity of the patient
Give an explanation and reassurance
Check the patient is not pregnant
Large opacities e.g. breast prosthesis, buckles, medallions should
be removed
Recent radiograph of the area may be required
    e.g. Lung scan — chest radiograph.

Other considerations

Radioactivity

After the injection, patients should not sit near pregnant women or
young children because of the radiation hazard
A separate waiting room may be required
In certain examinations nursing mothers should not breast feed for
48 hours as their milk will be radioactive.

Contamination

Urine and vomit disposed of down the toilet
Linen marked plastic bags, and stored, the length of storage
depends on the radionuclide used.

Emptying bladder

Prior to imaging, fluids are encouraged as the radiopharmaceutical
is excreted via the kidney, and bladder uptake may obscure the
bony pelvis.

Diet

Biliary imaging and thyroid uptakes — patient starved overnight.

Drugs

Potassium perchlorate may be given to discharge the thyroid gland prior to the introduction of a radiopharmaceutical e.g. thyroid scans Certain thyroid medications are withdrawn prior to thyroid uptake examinations.

COMPUTERISED TOMOGRAPHY

General preparation

Check the identity of the patient
Give an explanation and reassure the patient
Remove opacities from the area of the examination.

Preparation for specific examinations

Brain scans

Large bandages may have to be removed
Anaesthetic may be required
Premedication may be required for young children.

Whole body scans

Claustrophobic patients will require additional reassurance
Consider placing patient in machine feet first
Patient may have a fear of the diagnosis (due to the association of the machine with the diagnosis of carcinoma)
Abdomen should be free from barium sulphate which has been administered during a barium meal or enema
Abdominal preparation may be required
Dilute sodium diatrizoate and meglumine diatrizoate or dilute barium sulphate suspension (225 ml in 900 ml water) may be given to outline the gasto-intestinal tract
Intravenous contrast agents can be administered to demonstrate the circulatory system and therefore a check on patient allergies should be made.

Guided biopsies

Sterile procedure

Premedication given
Procedure usually under local anaesthetic.

NUCLEAR MAGNETIC RESONANCE

General preparation

Check the identity of the patient
Give explanation and reassure the patient because:
  It is important to reduce movement due to the length of the scan
  time
  Some patients have problems with claustrophobia
Sedation may be used with young children
Remove all objects affected by magnetism from the room i.e. iron-based objects.
Remove opacities from the area of the examination
Aneurism clips and metal implants may cause artifact problems
Check the patient does not have a pacemaker — as this will be affected by the magnetic field
Check the patient does not have a history of epilepsy — the magnetic field may cause a fit
Check the patient does not have a history of myocardial infarction
Dimeglumine gadopentetate can be used to enhance intracranial and spinal lesions. This should not be used with patients under 18 years or during pregnancy.

10. Patient preparation — radiotherapy; care of radiation reactions

INTRODUCTION

Advancing radiation treatment techniques are designed to spare normal tissue wherever possible, whilst delivering a high tumour dose to a prescribed area.

Unfortunately, some irradiation of normal cells is unavoidable and these produce 'side effects'.

To alleviate the worries caused to the patients by these side effects, the radiotherapy team of radiographers, radiotherapists and nursing staff should be able to give a clear explanation to these patients and be able to minimise the side effects with a high standard of treatment and nursing care.

The use of megavoltage photon beams provides some degree of protection to the skin as the maximum dose occurs at a depth below the skin surface. However, clinically important skin reactions are still a common problem in radiotherapy departments.

STAGES OF ACUTE SKIN REACTIONS

First degree following a single dose to the skin of 750–1000 cGy
Erythema — reddening of the skin, caused by congestion of the blood vessels (temporary)
Epilation

Second degree following a single dose to the skin of 1000–1500 cGy
Bright erythema
Epilation
Arrest of sweat production
Erythema starts to disappear when basal cells start to regenerate
Peeling off of extra dead cells from the surface — dry desquamation.

Third degree following a single radiation dose to the skin of 1500–
2000 cGy
   3250 cGy in 5 treatments over 1 week
   5000 cGy in 20 treatments over 4 weeks
Deep erythema
Loss of epithelial cell structure
Release of intra/extra cellular fluid — moist desquamation, dries
with scab formation
Permanent epilation
Arrest of sweat production (may be permanent)
All of the above are 'normal' reactions.

Fourth degree
Radiation necrosis — can be caused by radiation overdosage
Breakdown of epidermis and dermis
Destruction of blood vessels
Damage to sensory nerve endings therefore necrotic area very
painful
Healing delayed or non-existent.

LATE CHANGES FOLLOWING ACUTE SKIN REACTIONS

Pigmentation

Due to increased synthesis of melanin
Increased number of melanocytes
Migration of melanocytes within the epidermis.

Telangiectasia

Dilatation of terminal capillaries to compensate for artery impairment around the irradiated area. (Can occur anywhere in the body).

Ischaemia

Destruction of blood vessels leading to a reduced blood supply to
the skin (and other organs)
Makes subsequent healing in the area difficult.

Fibrosis

Skin loses elasticity
Thickening can occur

Total loss of blood supply leads to necrosis
The irradiated skin will always be more susceptible to damage and
the patient must be told of care needed for this area.
  No exposure to intense sunlight, wind or cold
  Prevent the area from receiving friction/irritants which could
  precipitate skin breakdown.

CARE OF THE PATIENT FOLLOWING RADIOTHERAPY

Explain the anticipated reaction
Treatment area kept free from friction e.g.
  No rubbing the skin
  No shaving
  No tight clothing around the treatment area.
  During the treatment period the area may be dusted with a light
chalk powder (ZeaSORB) which often helps to keep the skin more
comfortable against the patient's clothing. Contraindicated are
powders containing metallic oxides as the presence of these metals
would create a characteristic radiation which would add to the skin
dose
Any dressing within the treatment area should be kept in place by
Netalast bandage or a nonmetallic tape such as Micropore tape.
Watch for a reaction from an exit dose on megavoltage units
For a skin reaction proceeding to moist desquamation
  Discontinue the powdering
  Dressings to cover the area when in a public place to help prevent
  infecting the area.

For itchy reactions

Crotamiton lotion (contraindicated for patients with dermatitis).

Painful reactions

Hydrocortisone cream (POM). Stop if reaction breaks down.

Washing the affected skin

This advice will depend upon the degree of reaction present. However, psychologically, it is better for the patients to wash. Use tepid
water and non-perfumed soap.

REACTIONS IN THE ORAL CAVITY

Arising following irradiation of the oral cavity
   High dose radiotherapy to an oral tumour treating to a target
   dose (TD) of 6000 cGy in 25 treatments over 5 weeks
   Patients receiving radiotherapy to the oral cavity/cervical lymph
   nodes under the CHART regime (continuous, hyperfractionated,
   accelerated radiotherapy).
The oral cavity and the pharynx are lined with mucous membrane
which is highly sensitive to radiation.

1st stage

Inflammation of the membrane — mucositis
Goblet cells cease to function
Mouth becomes sore and dry

2nd stage

Formation of a protective white membrane — from fluid released
from damaged cells
Fluid mixes with dead surface cells

3rd stage

Membrane adheres to underlying damaged tissue, repair begins
Radiation effects on the salivary glands adds to the dryness
Saliva contains a bacteriostatic agent which helps prevent the mouth
from becoming infected

Care of the patient

Before radiotherapy commences all patients, with their own teeth,
should have them inspected. Any carious teeth should be removed
before treatment
Good dental and oral hygiene should be encouraged
Radiotherapy may precipitate dental decay due to:
   Reduction in the blood supply to the teeth
   Exposure of the tooth root if the radiation causes gum shrinkage
   Risk of infection due to impairment of the salivary glands
   Some degree of protection can be afforded by bridging the teeth
   with a protective cap during the treatment and reaction period.

Patients suffering from dysphagia

Benzocaine mucilage before meals is an effective analgesic.
Use of frequent mouthwashes e.g. glycerin and thymol
Gentle teeth cleaning
Antiseptic mouthwashes may be substituted if infection is present
e.g. povidone-iodine (an iodine-based antiseptic)
Fungal infections can be prevented by an oral suspension e.g. containing nystatin
Food may be liquidised, nothing too hot or spicy
Alcoholic spirits should be avoided

Anorexia will be a problem because of the soreness and lack of or altered taste due to impairment of the taste buds.

REACTIONS OF THE BOWEL

The most sensitive area of the bowel to radiation is the small intestine
    Consists of a lining of columnar epithelium
    Goblet cells are scattered among the epithelial cells
    Surface is covered by millions of projections called villi which greatly increase the surface area
    The generative cells for epithelial replacement are found at the base of the villi — the crypts.

Crypts

Radiation causes the cells to swell up and disintegrate
Debris collects in them.

Villi

Shorten because of lack of replacement cells
Total destruction of a large area of intestinal villi would lead to death of the patient through dehydration and loss of electrolytes
Radiation doses for malignant disease in the abdomen and pelvis are not sufficient to cause total and irreversible damage, villi regeneration quickly returns.

Diarrhoea

May occur hours after commencement of treatment indicating the speed with which the absorbing properties of the bowel are affected.

Care of the patient

The patient should be advised that the reactions are normal.

For the treatment of the diarrhoea

Attention to diet — resist all foods which loosen the stools
High fluid intake — In patients will have a fluid balance chart
Troublesome diarrhoea responds to
    Codeine phosphate
    Loperamide

Tenesmus

Patient may complain of severe spasmodic abdominal cramps
(tenesmus) which arises due to acute inflammation in the treatment
area
Peristalsis is affected leading to constipation above the inflamed
area
Pethidine will relieve the pain
It is expected that patients experiencing acute bowel reactions will
be nursed on the radiotherapy ward.

EPILATION

This is loss of hair — temporary below a skin dose causing
    moist desquamation, permanent at a skin dose causing moist
    desquamation
    Radiotherapy — Epilation only occurs within the treatment and
exit dose areas.
    Chemotherapy — Epilation caused by some drugs is a general effect which occurs because of the effect on the regenerating cells of
the hair in the hair bulb. If there is total destruction of these cells
permanent epilation will result.
    Psychologically, epilation is extremely damaging for many patients.
If patients are expected to have total hair loss over a period of time,
they should be referred to the NHS wig specialist before the hair
loss occurs

RADIATION EFFECTS ON THE BONE MARROW

Bone marrow is highly sensitive to radiation

Red bone marrow

Contains the haemopoeitic tissue
Large field irradiation significantly affects blood cell production
In adult life red bone marrow is found in the:
    sternum
    iliac crests
    skull
    upper end of humeri
    upper end of femori
    scapulae
    clavicles
    vertebrae

Blood counts

A drop in peripheral platelet and white cell counts may be noticeable following only a few treatment sessions.
White cells have a relatively short life span — average 7 days.
Red cells with a life span of 120 days are not affected so rapidly.
Patients with falling blood counts should be sent for regular blood counts, daily blood counts may be required.

Care of the patient

Leucopenia — reduced white cell count. Do not treat patients who have white blood counts below 2.0×10^9/litre — this leads to a reduced ability to cope with infections.

Patients should be warned of the risks of going to public places like theatres, should avoid people with diagnosed infections and should report any ill health or temperature rise immediately.

Patients contracting infections should be treated with the appropriate antibiotics.

Thrombocytopenia — reduced platelet count. A count below 60×10^9/litre will lead to an increased risk of haemorrhage.

Purpura — haemorrhage of the skin and mucous membranes.

Anaemia

Reduction in the number of circulating red blood cells, the haemoglobin level is often below 9 g/dl.
May occur in malignant disease involving the bone marrow, in Hodgkin's Disease, hypersplenism and following prolonged haemorrhage.

Patients may complain of

Malaise
Lassitude
Headache
Amenorrhoea
Patients will appear pale.

Nursing care includes

Adequate rest
Care of the skin, mouth and teeth
Attention to diet
Antianaemic drugs — as prescribed by medical officer
A blood transfusion may be prescribed if haemoglobin falls below 9 g/dl.

RADIATION EFFECTS ON THE GONADS AND FETUS

Photon radiation doses as low as 10 cGy can cause fetal abortion in early pregnancy.

In later pregnancy when organogenesis is taking place, malformations may be seen in the newborn infant.

If it is necessary to irradiate a pregnant female, the fetus should be protected from the radiation.

Ovarian effects

In the early developing ovarian follicle, the oocyte and the granulosa cells are very radiosensitive.

Radiation effects on the ovaries depend on the dose received and the age of the female. The younger the woman, the greater the dose has to be to achieve a particular effect. Deliberate suppression of ovarian function — a radiation induced menopause may be carried out for several reasons:

To suppress ovarian hormones in malignant disease which has a hormone dependency e.g. some breast cancers.
To suppress ovarian hormones associated with menstrual problems e.g. menorrhagia.
Indirect suppression may occur when irradiating the pelvis or abdomen for other malignant disease.

Care of the patient

Careful explanation of the effects to the patient and partner.
Warned that suppression is not an immediate effect and contraception should be continued, if necessary, for up to 18 months.
Consent form should be signed by patient, before commencement of treatment.
Patients may experience menopausal symptoms e.g. hot flushes, vaginal dryness following radiotherapy.
Diarrhoea may be a problem, depending on the area of treatment and the radiation dosage (see section on bowel reactions).

Testicular effects

Spermatogonia are very radiosensitive.
Permanent sterility has been known to occur at testicular doses of 500 cGy. However, sperm production after radiation therapy follows an unpredictable pattern.
The interstitial cells which produce testosterone are not affected at these dose levels.

Care of the patient

Patients should be told of the side effects of radiation to the testicles.
Provision for the use of a sperm bank for these patients.

Genetic mutations

Very low doses, radiation levels too low to affect mitosis in the gonads, change the genetic structure, leading to genetic mutations in any offspring. It is therefore important for student radiographers to understand how to prevent the ovaries and testes from receiving radiation which could lead to genetic mutation in later generations. Therefore radiotherapy for the treatment of non-malignant disease in the younger generation is only used if other forms of treatment have proved unsuccessful.

RADIATION EFFECTS ON THE EYE

May be seen following radiotherapy to the eye:
    primary treatment for an orbital tumour or
    carcinoma of the antrum, involving the orbit
Retina is not radiosensitive at radiotherapy dosages.
Cornea, conjunctiva and the lens are more radiosensitive.
Eyelids are affected in the same way as the skin.

Conjunctiva

Conjunctival hyperaemia occurs soon after radiotherapy commences.
Swelling may lead to conjunctivitis, the columnar epithelium becomes keratinised.
Scarring may develop.

Care of the patient

To help prevent permanent damage, infection must be prevented with antibiotics e.g. gentamicin or chloramphenicol eye ointment

Lacrimal glands

Reduction or absence of secretions leads to 'dry eye' syndrome
May lead to keratitis, infection and ulceration.

Care of the patient

Antibiotics prescribed to combat infection on the conjunctiva
Artificial tear solutions.

Cornea

Corneal oedema and keratitis, worsened if lacrimal glands are affected.

Care of the patient

Keep inflammation to a minimum
Antibiotics prescribed.

The ocular lens

X and gamma radiation doses of more than 200 cGy to the lens can cause cataract formation.

Radiation affects mitotic activity in the germinative zone of lens epithelium.

Epithelial cells differentiate into lens fibres, in the posterior capsule, swell up to form large, balloon-like cells, developing into cataracts.

The damaged cells migrate to region of posterior pole and increase in size.

If the damaged area cannot be limited by repair processes, the opacity will involve the whole lens.

Care of the patient

The obvious treatment is prevention.

The dose to the lens is minimised by accurate beam direction and shielding of the lens with the appropriate thickness of lead.

Use may be made of the 'build-up' region on megavoltage which may allow the maximum dose to be delivered posterior to the lens.

If cataracts do appear, the only treatment is surgical resection.

RADIATION SICKNESS

A general reaction occurring during large field radiotherapy to widespread or bulky tumours.

These tumours may affect the patient with their own metabolic activities and by diversion of necessary nutrients to the tumour.

Following radiotherapy, these cellular, bulky tumours can produce excess nucleic acid, which needs to be excreted by the kidneys.

The radiotherapy will also affect normal tissues.

All the factors together produce a clinical picture of radiation sickness.

Care of the patient

Careful explanation should be given to the patient before treatment commences

Tiredness   —ensure plenty of rest

Nausea or vomiting   —antiemetics — pyridoxine hydrochloride
                                                (vitamin B6)

	prochlorperazine
	(Stemetil)
	domperidone
Anorexia	—small nourishing meals
	high fluid intake should be maintained

Headache/
general aches and pains—suitable analgesic.

SUMMARY

The above section on radiation reactions is by no means complete. It is intended to help student radiographers realise the need for a high standard of patient care if radiation side effects are to be kept to a minimum. Not included in this section are the effects of radiation on organs such as kidneys, lungs and the central nervous system, which are of no less importance. Radiographers need to understand how to minimise all radiation effects on all normal tissues, but this section is intended primarily to look at some of the radiation effects which occur during the course of radiotherapy, which then come under the care of the radiographer.

Further reading on this complex subject can be obtained in the following books:

Coggle J E 1971 Biological Effects of Radiation, Wykeham Publications, London and Winchester
Nias A H W 1988 Clinical Radiobiology, (2nd Ed), Churchill Livingstone, Edinburgh
Lerman S 1980 Radiant Energy and the Eye, Balliere Tindall, New York
Walter J, Miller H, Bomford C K 1979 A Short Textbook of Radiotherapy, Churchill Livingstone, Edinburgh
Lowry S 1974 Fundamentals of Radiation Therapy, English Universities Press Limited, London

CARE OF THE PATIENT DURING SPECIAL PROCEDURES

KNIFE BIOPSY

Bios — life
Opsis — vision

A knife biopsy is carried out to obtain a section of skin/ subcutaneous tissue for histological examination e.g. confirmation of diagnosis of a basal carcinoma of the skin, malignant skin deposits from a breast carcinoma.

If a small lesion is suspected of being a basal cell carcinoma the whole lesion can be completely excised either by a scalpel or a curette (excision biopsy).

Duties of the radiographer

To prepare the biopsy trolley
To care for the patient before, during and after the procedure
To assist the radiotherapist during the procedure

Trolley setting

Wash hands thoroughly, dry on a paper towel
Shelves and rails sprayed with disinfectant
Dried with a sterile towel
Attach bag for dirty swabs

Nonsterile equipment

On the bottom shelf place:
   Labelled specimen jar
   Receiver for soiled dressing
   Antiseptic sprays
   Adhesive tape
Wash hands, dry

Sterile equipment

This should be set out as near to the time of the biopsy as possible to prevent contamination of the equipment by an airborne route.
On the top shelf open a toilet and suture pack containing:
   Outer coverings and dressing towels
   Gallipots, 2, which should contain an antiseptic e.g. chlorhexadine for skin disinfection, and 1 containing sterile water for rinsing any equipment such as the anaesthetic capsule which may have been sterilised in chlorhexadine
   Gauze swabs and cotton wool balls.
   Selection of forceps: Spencer Wells
                      dissecting forceps
   Scalpel or curette (previously sterilised)
   Suture needle and silk
   Scissors

Syringe, needle and local anaesthetic (lignocaine)
Surgeons gloves (disposable)
The top of the trolley is covered with a sterile towel.

Patient care

Reassure the nervous patient
Help the patient onto the couch
Remove any clothing as necessary from the patient
Explain the procedure to the patient
Reassure the patient throughout the procedure
Assist with the after-care of the patient
    Check that the dressing is secure
    Arrange further appointments for follow up and for the removal
of any stitches.

The radiographer should also

Check that the form accompanying the biopsy specimen has been
completed by the radiotherapist and that it accompanies the
specimen which is also correctly labelled
Tidy the room afterwards.

THE PATHOLOGY FORM

A form requesting a pathological report on a specimen sent for
examination.
For example:
    Specimen — blood
    Request — blood count
    Specimen — skin and underlying tissue
    Request — histology
The form should include the following details
    Hospital
    Department or ward
    Medical Officer in charge of the patient
    Nature of specimen
    Examination requested
    Clinical data of the patient
    Present treatment
Patient details
    Hospital number

Surname
Forenames
Sex
Age
Ethnic origin
Date and time specimen was taken
Signature of the Medical Officer
Pathology
Report number
Date the specimen was received
Time the specimen was received
Full pathology report
2 copies
1 sent to the Medical Officer
1 retained in pathology department.

TROLLEY SETTING FOR A PELVIC EXAMINATION

This is a socially clean procedure (not sterile)
Trolley cleaned with antiseptic solution
Dried
Covered with a clean disposable towel

Articles placed on the trolley

Gloves
Lubricant
Sponge holding forceps
Vulsellum forceps
Vaginal speculum
Proctoscope (if rectal examination is needed)
Gallipot with antiseptic solution
Swabs
Lamp
Receiver for soiled dressings and instruments
Spatula
Glass slides and cover slips
Sanitary towel.

Duties of the radiographer

Prepare the trolley

Explain procedure to the patient
Assist patient with undressing and positioning
Reassure patient during the procedure
Act as chaperone for male medical staff
Arrange patient appointment and further transport
Tidy the room.

TROLLEY SETTING FOR AN INDIRECT LARYNGOSCOPY

This is an indirect inspection of the larynx which is done during a
course of radical radiotherapy to the larynx so that the radiation
reaction can be assessed, and at follow up appointments to check
on the results of the radiotherapy e.g. radiation reactions, presence
of infection, tumour response
This is a clean procedure (not sterile).

Requirements

Large instrument tray with:
   Laryngeal mirror
   Spatula
   Paper towels and gauze swabs
   Finger stalls
Also required are:
   Benzocaine spray (to anaesthetise the throat)
   Spirit lamp and matches (to warm the laryngeal mirror)
   Bowl for dentures
   Mouth wash for patient
   Receiver for dirty swabs
   Head mirror — this is worn by the radiotherapist
      to reflect the light from behind the patient on to the laryngeal
      mirror in the throat.
If an infection is thought to be present the following are needed:
   Throat swab
   Labels
   Pathological request form

Duties of the radiographer

Prepare the trolley

Position the patient prior to the procedure
Assist the radiotherapist throughout the procedure
Reassure the patient throughout
Tidy the trolley afterwards
Lock away the benzocaine spray
Arrange transport if necessary
Arrange appointments if necessary
Check the forms if a throat swab has been taken.

TROLLEY SETTING FOR AN INJECTION OF RADIOACTIVE PHOSPHORUS (^{32}P)

An intravenous injection of ^{32}P can be given as part of the treatment of polycythaemia rubra vera.
Sterile procedure, therefore the trolley is prepared as described previously.
On the upper shelf place the following sterile equipment
  Dressing towel
  Gallipots containing — chlorhexadine for skin disinfection
  Syringe of appropriate size for the injection
  Selection of swabs and cotton wool balls
Lower shelf
  Tourniquet
  Selection of disposable needles
  Surgeons gloves (disposable) — prior to opening
  Plastic apron
  Dressings for the injection site following the procedure
  Receiver for dirty (non-contaminated) dressings
  Plastic bag or special receiver for contaminated articles
  Specially coated protective sheeting with an absorbing side and a waterproof side
  Radiation counter.

Duties of the radiographer

Prepare the trolley
Prepare the room — placing the absorbent sheeting in the appropriate places
Check that the correct amount of ^{32}P has been ordered and delivered

An intravenous dose of 150—220 megabecquerels (MBq) is usually the standard
Assist the patient into correct position
Assist the radiotherapist during the procedure
Release the tourniquet when the vein for injection has been located and the needle is in position
Reassure the patient throughout the procedure.

After the procedure has finished

Tidy the room
Remove the contaminated articles to the appropriate protection area
Check that the patient's wound has stopped bleeding
Check the room and staff for contamination using the geiger counter
Check patient for contamination (other than at the injection site)
Arrange for transport
Arrange a follow-up appointment
Store unused ^{32}P in the protected area.

CARE OF THE PATIENT UNDERGOING CHEMOTHERAPY

INTRODUCTION

Cytotoxic drugs now play a major role in the treatment of malignant disease. Radiographers have in their care, patients undergoing chemotherapy and radiotherapy and therefore need to understand the side effects of both of these treatments if the patient is to receive the best care and attention.

To discuss all cytotoxic drugs and their side effects would be impossible and probably soon out of date. The aim, therefore, is to discuss the common side effects of cytotoxic therapy.

Each drug has individual toxic actions but one property is common to all of them and that is they are unable to distinguish between normal and malignant cells. This means that when a cytotoxic drug is in the body it will attack all cells and so it is necessary to minimise the damage to the normal cells whilst enhancing the toxic effect on the malignant cells.

GROUPS OF CYTOTOXIC AGENTS

Alkylating agents

Mode of action within the cell

The drugs replace the hydrogen bond between the DNA bases with a hydrocarbon (alkylation). It is thought that this action prevents these base areas from acting as templates for new DNA replication.

Alkylation of enzymes in the cell prevents them from fulfilling their role in DNA replication.

Examples

Nitrogen mustard
Cyclophosphamide
Ifosfamide
Melphalan
Chlorambucil

Antimetabolites

Mode of action within the cell

Metabolites are incorporated into new proteins and nucleic acid prior to mitosis.

Antimetabolite cytotoxic drugs chemically resemble these metabolites and are taken into the nucleus. The cell is then incapable of protein synthesis, or forms protein not able to function as required by the cell.

Examples

Methotrexate   — prevents purine and pyrimidine synthesis
5 Fluorouracil   — prevents pyrimidine synthesis
Cytarabine   — prevents pyrimidine synthesis
6 Mercaptopurine   — prevents purine synthesis

NB. Purines and pyrimidines are essential constituents of DNA and RNA.

Compounds of biological origin

Mode of action within the cell

Not clear.

Thought to act in the early stage of cell division by interfering with RNA and DNA synthesis.

Examples

Vincristine
Vinblastine.

Antimitotic antibiotics

Mode of action within the cell

Attaches itself to a DNA molecule at the site where transfer RNA usually functions, preventing the DNA from reduplicating.

All the antibiotic cytotoxic drugs potentiate the action of radiotherapy leading to extreme skin reactions when both are used.

Examples

Actinomycin D
Mitomycin C
Doxorubican hydrochloride
Bleomycin.

Miscellaneous

Asparaginase — destroys all free asparagine in the body.

Asparagine is an amino acid essential to all cells. Malignant cells cannot make asparagine, therefore this drug exploits a biochemical difference between normal and malignant cells.

Value has proved limited because of severe toxicity and a rapid resistance to the drug.

Nitrosoureas — carmustine and lomustine.

Often classed as alkylating agents, but they also inhibit mitosis by blocking certain enzymes necessary for purine synthesis.

Cisplatin — thought to have action similar to alkylating agents, highly nephrotoxic.

Carboplatin — a newer platinum analogue, less nephrotoxicity.

GENERAL PRINCIPLES

Cytotoxic drugs may be used as:

A curative treatment

e.g. Chorioncarcinoma, a malignant tumour of the placenta, can be successfully treated in the early stages with methotrexate and actinomycin D.

An adjuvant to surgery/radiotherapy

e.g. Nephroblastoma of the kidney is now treated using a combination of surgery, radiotherapy and cytotoxic therapy, which has dramatically increased the survival rate.

A palliative treatment when other treatment methods have failed

e.g. Metastatic carcinoma of the breast when surgery, radiotherapy and hormone therapy have failed to control the disease.

GENERALISED SIDE EFFECTS FROM THE USE OF CYTOTOXIC THERAPY

Bone marrow depression

Some drugs cause an immediate drop in the blood count by affecting the cells already in the blood (limited effect).
Other drugs affect the stem cells in the bone marrow leading to delayed effects in the peripheral blood.
Leucopenia occurs first.
Life span of leucocytes averages 5 days, therefore the effects are seen in under a week.

Care of the patient

There is increased risk of contracting infection
Treatment is suspended if white cell count falls to 2.0×10^9/litre
Bone marrow is allowed to recover
Patients warned about the risk of infection
If white blood count drops very low following intensive treatment, the patient may have to be nursed in protective isolation
Pyrexia could indicate that infection is present
A broad spectrum antibiotic can be given until the infection has been identified.

Thrombocytopenia

A reduction of circulating blood platelets
Can be seen two weeks after the start of chemotherapy.

Care of the patient

Treatment is suspended if the platelet count falls to 50×10^9/litre
Patients warned of the risk of haemorrhage therefore male patients
advised to use electric razors
Problems with excessive menstruation ⎫
Sudden epistaxis ⎬ inform the Medical Officer
General body bruising ⎭

Erythrocytopenia

Not normally seen after cytotoxic therapy
Red blood cells have a life span of 120 days
Effects would not be seen for several months — meanwhile the
bone marrow should be recovering from the treatment
If the haemoglobin level is below 9 g/dl, a blood transfusion may
be given.

Epilation

Many drugs are capable of causing hair loss
Vincristine and adriamycin are particularly toxic to the hair follicles
Has the same psychological effect as with radiation induced hair
loss
Scalp hair is more sensitive to damage than other body hair
Regrowth readily occurs as the follicles quickly develop a resistance
to the drugs
It is necessary to provide wigs during the epilation period.

Gastrointestinal effects

Effects depend on the drugs used and the dose
Bleomycin and methotrexate cause soreness of the mucosal lining
of the mouth and pharynx leading to painful ulceration.

Care of the patient

Glycerin and thymol mouthwashes

Careful use of toothbrushes
Benzocaine emulsion given before meals
Attention to diet — soft, bland food
High fluid intake
For infections — antibiotic therapy
If thrush develops — nystatin suspension
Dental caries may be precipitated by cytotoxic therapy
Carious teeth should be removed beforehand
Nausea and vomiting are often a problem
Some drugs irritate the gastric lining e.g. carmustine
Some stimulate the vomiting centre in the brain e.g. nitrogen mustard
Patients have been known to vomit at the thought of having cytotoxic therapy
Antiemetics should be prescribed
A light diet should be advised
Diarrhoea is controlled with the appropriate drugs e.g. loperamide capsules
A high fluid intake is recommended.

Reproductive system

Many cytotoxic drugs suppress spermatogenesis and oogenesis
Alkylating agents are particularly toxic
Provision of sperm banks for the male patients
Female patients should be warned of irregular menstrual cycle.

Genetic mutations

The effect of cytotoxic therapy on the chromosomes is not fully understood
Effects may become more apparent with increasing use of cytotoxic therapy and an increase in the number of long-term survivors
During pregnancy it is thought unwise to give treatment during the first 3 months and methotrexate and the alkylating agents are absolutely contraindicated during this period
Long-term use of nitrogen mustard may be linked to secondary carcinogenesis.

Hyperuricaemia

Excess uric acid in the blood stream

Caused by breakdown of purine bases of DNA

Uric acid cannot be destroyed in the body, therefore it must be excreted

Toxic effects of excess uric acid includes renal damage and swollen joints (gout)

Occurs where there has been rapid breakdown of a large number of tumour cells due to chemotherapy or radiotherapy

Treatment — allopurinol converts the uric acid into a less toxic form for excretion.

Immunosuppression

Majority of cytotoxic drugs are known to suppress the body's immune response system

Patients are more susceptible to infections and can cope less readily with any invading pathogen

It is thought that a long-term effect is the risk of developing a new malignancy because of the immunosuppression

This may prove to be important as more patients are treated and survive for many years.

11. Drugs

INTRODUCTION

Patients attending an imaging or radiotherapy department may be receiving a variety of drugs. Although drug prescribing is the province of the medical staff, radiographers should have enough knowledge to understand the effects of drugs and what may happen if the patient has forgotten to take a particular drug or has taken too much in error.

This section is intended as a brief outline of the complex data of drug classification and gives examples of each category. Drugs used in the departments should be familiar to all staff and their desired effects and side effects understood. Student radiographers should know the principles behind the use of addictive drugs and the importance of following the strict procedures for the ordering, storage and administration of these drugs.

It is anticipated that students will obtain the widest experience of the use of drugs during their ward experience.

Drugs are substances used for medicinal purposes, they can be a source of danger to the patient if taken in sufficient quantity.

LAWS CONTROLLING DRUGS

Medicines Act (111) 1968

Regulates all aspects of the production and distribution of drugs and medicines whether for human or animal use.

The drugs covered under this act are classified as follows:

General Sale List medicines (GSL)

Drugs on this list can be sold in such places as supermarkets, but only in specific conditions e.g. some analgesics if they are prepacked and the pack contains not more than 25 tablets. They may not be sold from market stalls or vending machines.

Examples of drugs covered — common remedies for colds and coughs.

Pharmacy medicines (P)

There is no published list but this covers any drug not on the General Sale List or the Prescription Only Medicines (POM) list although some may contain POMs but at set strengths or doses. The drugs are under partial control and may only be sold if a pharmacist is present. The pharmacist can then advise when and how to use the drugs, and, if necessary, on any side effects which may occur.

Example of drugs covered — insulin.

Prescription Only medicines (POM)

Drugs on this list must have a written prescription, signed and dated in indelible ink, by a doctor or dentist. The full name and address of the patient and their age if under 12 years must be included.

Examples of drugs covered — cardiac drugs, chemotherapy drugs, antibiotics.

Misuse of Drugs Act 1971

Controls the manufacture, supply and possession of controlled drugs.

Misuse of Drugs Regulations 1985

Defines the people who are authorised to supply and possess controlled drugs and outlines the prescribing and record keeping procedures. The drugs are divided into 5 catagories:

Controlled Drugs CD (Lic.) — Schedule 1

Drugs for research purposes only
  e.g. hallucinogens

Controlled Drugs CD — Schedule 2

Drugs subject to full control and can be prescribed. Receipts and supplies must be recorded and special storage facilities are required
  e.g. morphine, amphetamine

Controlled Drugs CD No Register — Schedule 3

Drugs subject to full control and can be prescribed. Records do not have to be kept but invoices are kept for 2 years
  e.g. some barbiturates

Controlled Drugs CD (Benz) — Schedule 4

Subject to minimal control
  e.g. diazepam

Controlled Drugs CD (Inv) — Schedule 5

Drugs and strengths of drugs not normally considered to be high risk.

CONTAINERS AND LABELS

Containers

Can be
  Coloured bottle with child-proof lids
  Ampoules
  Bottles with rubber tops, the contents are removed with a syringe and needle, after the top has been cleaned with a sterile solution
  Ridged bottles — always contain poisons which are not for internal use.

Labels

Must be
  Indelible
  In English.
Must state
  Name, form and strength of drug
  Name of the patient
  Directions for use

Name and address of the supplier
Keep out of reach of children
Date
Cautions and additional advice.

UNITS OF MEASUREMENT

Milligrams   — mg
Grams   — g
Millilitres   — ml
Litres   — l
Weight/volume   — % strength

ADMINISTRATION

All drugs should be checked against the name of the patient:
    When the drug is removed from the cupboard
    When measuring the dose of the drug
    Before giving the drug to the patient.

By mouth

For each patient check the prescription, drug, dose and strength.

Medicine

Shake the bottle (unless stated otherwise)
Remove the stopper or screw cap
Hold with the label uppermost
Pour into the glass at eye level
Ensure the patient takes the drug.

Tablets

Check the number of tablets
Place the tablets in a container — no touch technique
Ensure the patient takes the tablets
In both cases record that the drug has been taken.

Disadvantages of the oral method

The patient may refuse to swallow the drug

The drug is only partially absorbed
The drug may irritate the stomach causing vomiting/diarrhoea.

Per rectum

For each patient check the prescription, drug, dose and strength.
The drug may be in the form of:
   Suppositories e.g. bisacodyl
   Enemas e.g. barium sulphate.

Inhalation

For each patient check the prescription, drug, dose and strength.
The drug may be in the form of vapour, liquid, gas, often used for
respiratory tract infections.
   For example, corticosteroid drugs for asthma e.g. betamethasone
            valerate,
            anaesthetic gases e.g. nitrous oxide

Injection

Sterile procedure
For each patient check the prescription, drug, dose and strength.

Trolley setting

Disposable cannula
         syringe
         needle.
Drug
Skin cleanser
Adhesive dressing
Bag for dirty swabs
Sharps box for needles and empty ampoules
Emergency drugs
alo Arm support
Tourniquet may be required.

Intravenous injection

The drug may only be administered by a doctor, or a member of
staff who has received additional training, if this route is used.

Reasons for the route

Quick acting in an emergency

Drug introduced into the circulatory system e.g. for diagnostic purposes

Anaesthetics may be introduced.

Sites

Midcubital vein of the forearm

Scalp veins.

Container

Ampoules.

Method

Explain the procedure to the patient

Reassure the patient

Show the doctor the ampoule prior to opening it

To check:

   Correct drug, type, strength

   Contents clear, not cloudy

   The expiry date

Apply the tourniquet

Support the arm

Clean the skin

Ask the patient to open and close their hand — to distend the veins in the elbow region

The sterile needle is inserted

Release the tourniquet prior to the injection.

After the injection

Apply swab and digital pressure to the puncture site

Apply an adhesive dressing

Dispose of the needle and ampoule in the sharps box

Dispose of the syringe and swabs

Put away the rest of the equipment.

Infusion

Allows the administration of large quantities of fluid, via a 'giving set' (Fig. 11.1) which controls the rate of flow, the solution may be given over a period of between 30 minutes and several days depending on the drug used.

For accurate monitoring of flow rate, electronically controlled drip feeders can be used. These monitor flow rate and will give an audible/visible signal if flow rate changes.

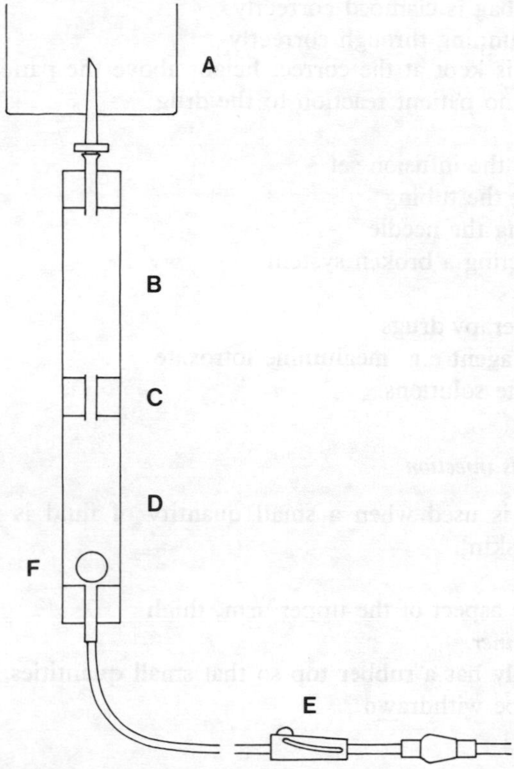

Fig. 11.1 Drip infusion set
A — Drug in solution in a plastic container
B — Filter chamber (removes solids)
C — Drip chamber (allows drip rate to be counted)
D — Float chamber
E — Flow control
F — Float ball (closes exit if chamber empty, to prevent air entering patient)

Site
Superficial veins — dorsum of hand, wrist
Containers
Bottle, bag
Method
See intravenous injection.

Care of the infusion set

   Ensure
   No contamination of the apparatus
   No air bubbles in the tubing

Infusion bag is clamped correctly
Drip is running through correctly
The bag is kept at the correct height above the patient
There is no patient reaction to the drug
Avoid
Straining the infusion set
Trapping the tubing
Dislodging the needle
Reconnecting a broken system
Examples
Chemotherapy drugs
Contrast agent e.g. meglumine iotroxate
Electrolyte solutions.

Subcutaneous injection

This route is used when a small quantity of fluid is introduced 'under the skin'.

Sites
Outer aspect of the upper arm, thigh
Container
Usually has a rubber top so that small quantities
may be withdrawn

Method
Explain the procedure to the patient
Reassure the patient
Wipe the bottle top with alcohol swab
Check and withdraw the required quantity of the drug
Change the needle
Swab the skin
Administer and record that the injection has been given
Examples
Adrenaline, insulin

Intramuscular injection

This route is used when large quantities of fluid are introduced.

Sites
Outer aspect of the shoulder
Antero-lateral aspect of the upper thigh
Upper, outer aspect of the buttocks

Container
Ampoules
Method
Explain the procedure to the patient
Reassure the patient
Check and open the ampoule, using a sterile swab to hold the top
Using a cannula, withdraw the drug
Replace the cannula with a needle
Swab the skin
Administer and record.
Examples
Penicillin, morphine, atropine.

CONTROLLED DRUGS

These must be kept in a locked cupboard, inside another locked cupboard, a red light may indicate when the door is open. The cupboard should be situated away from patients and the public in a cool, dry place. Designated key holders hold the keys, each person holding the key for 1 cupboard. 2 people must witness that the drug has been administered, 1 of whom must be a doctor or a Registered nurse.

Procedure

Collect the written prescription and the record book
Check that the patient has not already taken the prescribed dose of the drug
Select the drug and check the contents with the total in the book
Check the dose and the drug remaining in the container and the expiry date
Relock the drugs cupboard
Enter patient's name, dose of drug and the date given in the record book
Take the prescription and the drugs to the patient and recheck the quantity and the drug
Administer the drug to the patient
Enter the exact time of administration in the book
Both witnesses sign the book
   NB. Out of date drugs and those with illegible labels should be returned to the pharmacy.

DRUGS FOR PATIENT PREPARATION FOR DIAGNOSTIC EXAMINATIONS

Laxatives — aperients and suppositories used for bowel preparation
Sedatives — used to calm the patient
Premedications — used to relax the patient and reduce secretions prior to a general anaesthetic, may reduce postoperative vomiting
Local anaesthetic — used to stop sensation in a localised area
Analgesics — used to reduce pain
Contrast agents — used to outline organs in radiography.

RESUSCITATION DRUGS

Analeptic drugs — respiratory stimulants
Antihistamines — reduce allergic reactions
Examples of resuscitation drugs:
    Adrenaline — for cardiac arrest, raises blood pressure, will increase heart rate
    Atropine — for sinus bradycardia
    Lignocaine — for ventricular arrhythmias
    Hydrocortisone sodium succinate — reduces bronchospasm
    Digoxin — regulates heart action
    Isoprenaline — increases heart rate
    Frusemide — for oedema
    Chlorpheniramine maleate — antihistamine, anaphylactic shock.

ANAESTHETIC GASES

Nitrous oxide — cylinder is blue (anaesthetic)
Carbon dioxide — cylinder is grey (respiratory stimulant)
Entonox (oxygen and nitrous oxide) — cylinder is blue with a white and blue top (anaesthetic)
Oxygen — cylinder is black with a white cuff.

CONTRAST AGENTS

Air
Carbon dioxide
Barium sulphate
Iodine-based compounds.

12. Radiographic contrast agents

INTRODUCTION

During the course of their work, student radiographers will come into contact with many types of contrast agents, but because of individual radiological preferences, and the number of agents available, students may find that other agents or dosages are used in the departments in which they work. For the safety of the patient and the success of the examination, it is important that students understand the contraindications for the various contrast agents and to know why the specific agents are used.

Contrast agents are substances which can be used to demonstrate organs, vessels and parts of the body more clearly.

PRINCIPLES OF ACTION OF RADIOGRAPHIC CONTRAST AGENTS

As the atomic weights (total weight of protons and neutrons) of substances vary, the rate of absorption of X-radiation also varies.

The denser the substance the more the radiation is attenuated. Contrast agents may be of 2 types:

Negative — have a low atomic weight and therefore provide a negative contrast on the film as they absorb very little radiation.

Positive — have a high atomic weight and therefore provide a positive contrast on the film as they absorb most of the radiation.

NEGATIVE CONTRAST AGENTS

Air

This may be introduced by the patient e.g.

Chest radiographs — taken on inspiration, air in the lungs gives good tissue detail.

Valsalva manoeuvre — forced expiration on a closed glottis (alternative, asking the patient to breathe out, holding the air in the cheeks). Outlines the trachea.

Air or oxygen

Both gases can be retained by the body for a long period of time
Used if tomography is required
There is a danger of gas embolism forming
Air is introduced through a sterile swab to filter it.
e.g. Arthrography 30–40 ml of air or oxygen.
If gas embolism occurs
    Patient is placed on their left side
    The head is lowered
    Oxygen is given under positive pressure
    Cardiac arrest may occur, if so, cardiac massage is performed
    Patient must not sit up for several hours.

Carbon dioxide

Less risk of gas embolism
Rapidly absorbed (within 45 minutes)
e.g. *Barium meals* — to provide a double contrast with the barium
Can be in tablet, liquid, powder, or the carbon dioxide is ready mixed with the barium sulphate.

POSITIVE CONTRAST AGENTS

Barium sulphate

Introduced orally or per rectum.

Contraindications

Suspected fistula or sinus — because the barium sulphate is not absorbed by the body
Sometimes contraindicated prior to surgery — because the barium sulphate is not absorbed by the body.

Additives

Flavouring — makes the agent more palatable for children

Drugs

Hyoscine-N-Butylbromide — 20 mg given intravenously enables the stomach/colon to be examined free of muscle spasm
Metoclopromide — 10 mg given intravenously to co-ordinate peristaltic movement and therefore aids gastric emptying.

Iodine compounds

Non-ionic

Non-ionic contrast agents are most commonly used.

Advantages over ionic contrast agents

They do not dissociate in water
Risk of minor allergic reactions is reduced
Rapidly excreted via the kidneys
Lower viscosity
Lower osmolarity.

Disadvantages

Expensive
May provoke anaphylactic reactions.

Precautions

Store the agent correctly, usually at room temperature away from sunlight
Check if the patient has any history of allergy/asthma/hay fever/bronchitis
Have full resuscitation facilities available
Give drugs at body temperature
Manufacturer's doses should not be exceeded

Contraindications

Patient may have an allergy to iodine
If the patient has poor liver or renal function do not dehydrate
If the patient is a diabetic with high serum creatinine, above 500 μmol/l, they should not be examined.

Examples of non-ionic agents

Iohexol
Iopamidol
Iopromide
Ioxaglate.

Ionic agents

As these have a higher risk of patient reaction it is advisable, for medico-legal reasons, that they should only be used if no other agent is available and on low risk patients.

Examples of ionic agents

Sodium diatrizoate and meglumine diatrizoate
Calcium ipodate
Meglumine iotroxate.

It is suggested that a list of examinations, contrast agents (both chemical names and trade names) and example dosages used in your department is made and updated every year so that you are familiar with the drugs available.

Dosage of contrast agents

Varies according to:
    Patient's age
                condition
                weight
    Method of introduction
    Examination being undertaken
    Molecular size of the medium
    Children — dose according to body weight

Administration of contrast agents

Record — date, time, type, concentration, batch number, total dose, if any reaction
Doctor — checks name and concentration
               introduces contrast agent
Observe — for signs of
               reaction.

Reactions to contrast agents

Minor reactions	*Treatment*
Warmth, metallic taste in mouth	Reassure patient
Nausea, retching, sneezing	
	Observe and reassure
	If severe:
	Antihistamine
	Adrenaline 0.5 ml 1:1000
	subcutaneously
Extravasation of contrast agent into soft tissue	Warm compress
	Hyaluronidase IV

Major reactions

Seek medical help
Oxygen may be required
Initiate resuscitation procedure if required.

Could include:
    Erythema, urticaria, oedema of larynx
    Convulsions, coma
    Pulmonary oedema
    Hypotensive shock
    Cardiac arrest
    Respiratory arrest
    Cerebral oedema.
In all instances record the information concerning
    Type of reaction
    Contrast agent, dose and batch number
    Drugs given.

13. First aid

INTRODUCTION

Patients attending hospital for investigation or treatment may also require first aid treatment for a medical condition or an accident. Relatives and other visitors could also require first aid treatment.

Radiographers caring for patients must be able to recognise the signs and symptoms of medical emergencies and initiate the appropriate first aid action.

The ability to recognise a medical emergency and arrange for prompt treatment may well save a patient's life but it is important that in doing so you do not put yourself in danger.

GENERAL PRINCIPLES OF FIRST AID

To sustain life
To prevent the condition from becoming worse
To promote patient recovery.

ACTION SEQUENCE

If possible send for assistance (but do not leave the patient alone).
Check to see if the patient
    is breathing
    has a heart beat
    is bleeding
    has any broken bones
    has any burns.
In all instances
    Send for medical aid as soon as possible
    Administer the appropriate first aid
      e.g. resuscitate
          arrest haemorrhage etc.
          (see later for specific details)

FIRST AID TREATMENT

Condition	Cause	Signs and symptoms	First aid treatment
Shock occurs when the cardio-vascular system is incapable of delivering oxygen and nutrients to the cells		Skin grey, cold, clammy Body temperature drops Muscles relax Pulse rate increases and is weak Respiration becomes rapid, shallow and sighing Nausea Lowered blood pressure Loss of consciousness	Establish and remove cause Reassure the patient Keep warm and comfortable Lie patient flat and raise the legs (unless contraindicated e.g. injured) Move gently Check airway (dentures) If vomiting place in the coma position
Cardiogenic shock When the action of the heart is impaired	Disease of heart muscles Cardiac injury Heart failure		
Hypovolemic (medical) shock Loss of circulating blood volume	Haemorrhage Vomiting Diarrhoea Severe burns		Replace fluids
Vasovagal (neurogenic) shock Loss of vascular tone and therefore dilatation of blood vessels	Severe pain Fright		Reassure the patient Keep warm and comfortable.
Anaphylactic shock	Allergic reaction		Adrenaline injected Check vital signs Resuscitate if required

	Signs	Treatment
Electric shock		
High voltage (up to 400 kV)	May include: Cardiac arrest, Respiratory failure, Burns, Fractures, Shock	**DO NOT TOUCH EVEN INDIRECTLY UNLESS THE PATIENT HAS BEEN THROWN AWAY FROM THE SOURCE** When isolated: Check airway — resuscitate if required; Check pulse — resuscitate if required; Treat: Bleeding, Fractures, Shock; Report cause
Low voltage (Domestic supply under 415 V)	see High voltage	Switch off current or break contact using an insulator e.g. a lead rubber apron. Check airway — resuscitate if required; Check pulse — resuscitate if required; Treat: Bleeding, Fractures, Shock; Report cause; Equipment safety check
Asphyxia A condition when no oxygen can be delivered to the body cells, therefore increase carbon dioxide tension	Obstruction Paralysis of the respiratory muscles Breathing a medium with no air e.g. carbon monoxide	Breathing rate increased, Cyanosis, Noisy breathing, dyspnoea, Loss of consciousness — Remove patient from the cause; Clear airway; Check airway — resuscitate if required; Place in coma position

Condition	Cause	Signs and symptoms	First aid treatment
Burns Classified according to area and depth	Dry heat e.g. fire electricity friction strong acids/alkalis	May include: Reddening of the skin Pain Blistering Destruction of skin and underlying tissue	Cover with dry, sterile dressing to reduce risk of infection Treat for shock Do not remove clothing
Scalds	Moist heat	see Burns	see Burns Immerse in cold water for 10 minutes, if possible Remove clothing from body to prevent further scalding
Cerebrovascular accident (stroke)	When blood supply to brain is disrupted	Severe headache Full pulse Confusion Unconsciousness Dribbling Paralysis Slurred speech Weakness, one side of body Pupils may be unequally dilated Incontinence Hot, dry skin	Conscious — Send for medical aid Supine, head and shoulders raised Loosen clothing Keep warm Check vital signs Reassure Unconscious — Recovery position Check vital signs

	Cause	Signs and symptoms	First aid
Fainting	Temporarily inadequate supply of blood to the brain	Skin pale and clammy Perspiration on forehead Dizziness Ringing in ears Tingling in fingers Unconsciousness Vital signs all present	Check airway Undo tight clothing Open windows Place head lower than feet Rub face and hands Give the patient a drink unless contraindicated
Convulsions Uncontrolled generalised movements which may be associated with loss of consciousness	Unknown	Twitching of limbs Cyanosis Stiffness Head and spine arched Breath held prior to the attack	Check airway Loosen tight clothing Fresh air
Epilepsy (Type of convulsion)	Brain tumour Metabolic disturbances		
Petit Mal	Usually only occurs in children	Unconsciousness (short time) Pale Glassy expression in eyes Patient unaware of its occurrence	None usually required

Condition	Cause	Signs and symptoms	First aid treatment
Grand Mal	May be associated with organic disease e.g. tumour	Patient may have an aura *Tonic phase* Unconsciousness Muscle spasm Cyanosis Hands & teeth clenched Respiration ceases Patient rigid May cry out *Clonic phase* 30–60 second Contraction/relaxation of muscles Saliva may 'froth' from the lips ½–2 minutes later relaxes Patient wakens exhausted Coma Sleeps Recovers consciousness May vomit	Clear space round patient Loosen clothing Remove spectacles Prevent patient from injuring themselves. When recovered allow to rest Do not send home unaccompanied
Jacksonian Epilepsy (focal epilepsy)	Brain tumour Encephalitis Following head injury	Patients starts twitching (toes and fingers first) Twitching continues over one side of body May/may not lose consciousness.	None usually required Usual care for unconscious patients

			Immediate medical treatment
Status epilepticus		Repeated convulsions. Patient does not regain consciousness between them	
Epistaxis	Trauma to nose Spontaneous high blood pressure	Bleeding from the nasal cavity	Sit patient, head forward Patient breathes through mouth Pinch nose for 10 minutes Loosen clothing round neck Patient should not blow nose
Foreign bodies	In the eye	Excessive watering	Cover with clean cloth Do not attempt to remove
	In the ear	? pain	Small quantities of oil may be poured in the ear
	In the nose	Snuffling Bleeding	Cover with a clean, dry dressing To arrest bleeding apply indirect pressure
Myocardial infarction (heart attack)	Arterial occlusion e.g. coronary thrombosis	Pain in chest (crushing) Pain down left arm Nausea/sweating/vomiting Anxiety/fear of dying Dyspnoea/cyanosis Pain not reduced with glyceryl trinitrate	Send for medical aid Check vital signs Reassure, to reduce anxiety Observe patient Do not leave alone Patient semi-recumbent Oxygen if dyspnoeic

Condition	Cause	Signs and symptoms	First aid treatment
Poisoning	Corrosive substance e.g. phenol	Burns on lips and mouth Pain Vomiting Shock Thirst	Water or milk to drink
	Instant e.g. mercury arsenic	Pain in abdomen Vomiting blood Diarrhoea Collapse	Emetic — if cause is certain Gastric lavage If collapsed, warm abdomen
	Hypnotic and Neurotic e.g. morphine barbiturates	Drowsiness Coma Slow respiration	Give emetic Gastric lavage Artificial respiration Doctor required to give drugs to counteract
	Convulsant e.g. strychnine	Restlessness Delirium Convulsions	Give emetic Gastric lavage Rest Doctor required to give drugs to counteract
	Carbon monoxide	See Asphyxia	See Asphyxia

After care of the patient

Observe their — colour
                  pulse
                  respiratory rate
                  level of consciousness
Always check for delayed shock.

After the emergency

Fill in an accident form or occurrence report form
Report the incident to the superintendent in charge of the department
Report to the ward manager if the patient is an In patient
Report to the clinic manager if the patient is an Out patient.

14. Resuscitation procedure

INTRODUCTION

Following a cardiac arrest, irreversible brain damage will occur if the brain is starved of oxygen for more than 3 minutes. Successful application of external cardiac massage and artificial respiration must have saved countless numbers of lives.

It is unacceptable for a patient to die or be permanently mentally retarded after a cardiac arrest because of a lack of knowledge on resuscitation procedures by radiographers.

This section outlines the resuscitation procedure which should be known by every member of staff and every student. It would be of great value if the students are able to receive practical instruction on a special resuscitation dummy.

Special cardiac arrest teams, in hospitals, can be summoned by telephone, their telephone number should be known by everyone.

In all instances

Never leave the patient

Send for help

Check pulse e.g. carotid pulse

Check respiratory rate

CARDIAC ARREST

This is the failure of the heart to maintain the blood circulation.

Causes of cardiac arrest

Ventricular fibrillation

Myocardial infarction

Severe electrolyte imbalance

Electrocution

Dangers

Brain damage occurs if circulatory supply is not restored within 3 minutes.

Signs and symptoms of cardiac arrest

Sudden collapse of the patient
No pulse (carotid or femoral)
Loss of consciousness — check state by speaking loudly
Cessation of breathing
Cyanosis
Dilating or dilated pupils (late sign)

Procedure

Send for the cardiac arrest team

EXPIRED AIR RESUSCITATION — MOUTH TO MOUTH METHOD

Clear patient's airway
Extend neck — head well back
Check for breathing
Pinch nose with one hand
Support chin with the other hand — jaw forward
Take a deep breath in, place mouth over patient's mouth forming a seal
Exhale slowly and gently for 1.5 seconds
Turn to watch chest inflate (if chest does not inflate there could be an obstruction)
After 2 breaths check for major pulse
If pulse present, continue mouth to mouth at a rate of 12/minute
If absent, start external cardiac compression

EXTERNAL CARDIAC COMPRESSION

If cardiac arrest witnessed

Precardiac percussion — sharp blow to lower end of sternum
Check major pulse as the blow may have started the heart

If cardiac arrest not witnessed

Place patient on a hard surface e.g. imaging table/treatment couch/floor
Place heel of one hand over the lower third of sternum midway between the sternal angle and the xiphisternum in the midline
Place the other hand over the first
Lace the fingers to lift the palms off the ribs
Keep arms straight and shoulders forward
For an adult, push sternum down 4–5 cm using weight of the trunk
For a baby, sternum is depressed 2.5 cm
For a young child, sternum is depressed 2.5–3.5 cm
Use regular, smooth pressure
Continue at a rate of 60/minute

Interspace ventilations and external chest compressions as follows

1 operator — 2 breaths to 15 compressions
2 operators — 1 breath to 5 compressions with no break
Check for return of heartbeat after first minute and then every 3 minutes.

ALTERNATIVE TECHNIQUES

To clear obstructed airway
Heimlich manoeuvre

DO NOT PRACTISE ON VOLUNTEERS
Lean patient forward
Stand behind patient, arms round waist
Make a fist and place in the midline below the xiphisternum
Hold fist with other hand
Jerk hands inwards and upwards
If unsuccessful, repeat

If Brook airway available

Check that the airway is clear
Insert airway into the patient's mouth over the tongue into the back of the patient's mouth
Pinch patient's nose

Expand the patient's lungs via the airway (one way valve ensures patient's exhaled air escapes via the exit port).

If mouth to mouth contraindicated

e.g. facial injuries
      persistent vomiting
      tracheostomy patient
      patient prone

Alternative methods are:
  Mouth to nose
  Holger-Nielson
  Emergency tracheostomy and oxygen

If oxygen is available

Insert oral airway into the patient's mouth
Inlet of Ambu-bag attached to the oxygen supply 10–15 litres/minute oxygen required
Patient's chin held forward
Mask over patient's mouth forming a seal
Bag squeezed at the rate of 12/minute.

After the arrival of the cardiac arrest team, the following actions may be initiated.

Defibrillation

Electrodes of defibrillator covered with gel pads
  1 placed below the right clavicle
  1 placed over the apex to the heart — 5th intercostal space
  Ensure nobody is touching the table/patient
  DC shock of 160 joules given (may be increased up to 400 joules).

Cardiac monitor

Patient attached to the monitor
Patient's cardiac rhythm can be observed.

Table 14.1 Examples of drugs which may be given in cases of cardiac arrest

Diagnosis	Drug
Cardiac arrest	Adrenaline 10 ml of 1:10 000
Acidosis due to lack of respiration	Infusion — 50 ml 8.4% sodium bicarbonate
Sinus bradycardia	Intravenous atropine 0.6 mg
Ventricular arrhythmias	Intravenous lignocaine 100 mg
Ventricular tachycardia	Procainamide 100 mg
Emergency anaphylactic reaction	Adrenaline 0.5 — 1 mg of 1:1000
When cardiac arrest is prolonged	Calcium gluconate 10 ml of 10%

15. Administration of oxygen

INTRODUCTION

Oxygen, either in cylinders or piped from the wall, is present in every imaging and radiotherapy department.

It is important that student radiographers are taught how to use the equipment competently to ensure, not only the safety of the patient, but of the staff and the department. It is necessary for the student radiographers to be able to identify the component parts of the equipment and to understand their function.

The rules regarding the storage of oxygen should be known and understood. The student radiographers should be able to care competently for a patient who is receiving oxygen and should be aware of the methods of oxygen administration available. There should be an awareness of the types of patients who may require oxygen and an understanding of the observations which need to be made for these patients. It is expected that students gain practical experience in this subject whilst under experienced supervision.

Oxygen is required when the patient's normal supply of oxygen to the tissue cells cannot be maintained

e.g. Respiratory failure
    Circulatory failure
    Inability of cells to combine with oxygen (carbon monoxide poisoning).

OXYGEN SUPPLY

Piped

The pipes are clearly marked with the word oxygen.

Cylinders (Fig. 15.1)

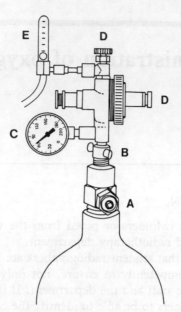

Fig. 15.1 A regulating valve on an oxygen cylinder
A — on/off switch from the cylinder
B — a locking nut for attachment to the cylinder
C — a pressure gauge — gives the pressure of oxygen in the cylinder when the
on/off switch is open
D — valves to control the oxygen supply from the regulator to the patient
E — a flowmeter to register the rate of flow to the patient

The cylinders are black with a white collar
  have oxygen or O_2 written on them
  are operated by a regulating valve.

MAINTENANCE AND CHECKING OF AN OXYGEN CYLINDER

The operator should check that the cylinder:
  Is easily accessible
  Is easily manoeuvered
  Is periodically checked for function
  Is kept clean
  Has a disk or tear off label indicating if it is full/empty/in use
  Has a valve spanner or key available
  Has the on/off valve open

Has tubing and masks readily available
NB. A full cylinder should always be available.

METHODS OF ADMINISTRATION

Oxygen is mixed with air before being given to a patient. If 100% oxygen is administered it could result in the patient suffering:
Pulmonary damage
Convulsions
Pain in the air sinuses and middle ear.

Masks — oral/nasal

Polymask — delivers 30–50% concentration of oxygen at 4 litres/minute (Fig. 15.2)
Disposable, light, a double bag with a wire frame, held in position by cords passed over the patient's head or ears. Oxygen passes in between the layers and enters the inner bag via two holes. There are small holes in the outer bag to allow the air to mix with the oxygen.

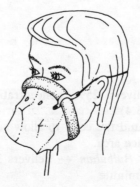

Fig. 15.2 *Polymask*

Edinburgh mask — delivers 35% concentration of oxygen at 3 litres/minute (Fig. 15.3)
Disposable, controlled low concentrations of oxygen administered. Air enters through the front opening. May have an attachment so that higher concentrations can be given.

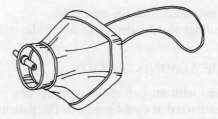

Fig. 15.3 *Edinburgh mask*

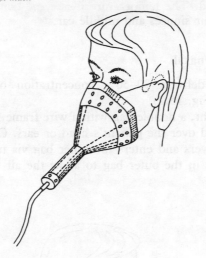

Fig. 15.4 *Ventimask*

Ventimask — delivers 25% concentration of oxygen at 4 litres/minute (Fig. 15.4)
Disposable, holes round the edge to allow air to enter, has a rigid base and a flexible face area.

Boothby, Lovelace, Bulbulian — delivers 30–40% concentration of oxygen at 4 litres/minute
Rubber mask and metal connector with a reservoir breathing bag. Patient's expired air mixes with the oxygen in the bag and the patient inspires air plus oxygen. Can be sterilised by autoclaving or gamma radiation.

Nasal tubes

Deliver 30–40% concentration of oxygen at 4 litres/minute
2 catheters are attached to a Y shaped tube, each is passed

2.5 cm along the floor of the nose. The oxygen is passed through a humidifier before being administered. Nasal tubes have the advantage that the patient can eat and drink with them in situ.

Oxygen tents

Deliver 40% concentration of oxygen at 10 litres/minute
Transparent plastic is attached to a metal frame and encloses the patient and bed. The temperature inside the tent is 18–21°C and to maintain this the oxygen is passed through ice, or a refrigeration unit. In some units the carbon dioxide is removed by passing the air through soda lime. There are plastic zip fasteners in the sides of the tent to allow nursing procedures to be carried out.

Ventilators

For a 70 kg man, 500 ml/breath, 12 breaths/minute, therefore 6000 ml/minute.

Artificial aid to breathing. Air is forced into the lungs via a mask/endotracheal tube/tracheostomy tube. The unit pumps air or oxygen rhythmically to and from the patient's lungs. Portable units are available. Observation should be made of the patient's colour, the chest movement and the tubing to ensure that it is not trapped.

Patient observations during oxygen administration

Patient's pulse and respiration rate
Colour of the patient
Signs of distress
Mask still in position
Tube supplying oxygen not kinked
Level of consciousness.

PRECAUTIONS

Oxygen itself will not burn, but it supports combustion. Therefore certain precautions must be taken to prevent fire or explosion.
Keep cylinders away from heat e.g. radiators
No smoking
No naked lights
No electric bells or heating pads
No mechanical toys — as they may cause sparks

Care when combing patient's hair — due to static
No nylon nightwear
Patient not rubbed with oil or spirit
No oil or grease used on the cylinder fittings
If the patient has to be radiographed,
   supply turned off
   speed and care during the examination
   turn on the supply again as soon as possible.

RECORDS

Any patient receiving oxygen should have a record kept of:
   The rate of flow
   Length of time administered
   Percentage of oxygen administered.

16. Tracheostomy and suction

INTRODUCTION

A patient with a tracheostomy needs special care and attention in the department. They need the assurance of knowing that the staff can competently care for them and should the tracheostomy tube begin to block there will be staff present to give assistance.

This is of particular importance to the radiotherapy staff who may be treating a patient with a tracheostomy for several weeks. If the treatment fields are in the region of the tracheostomy it is important that the students understand the importance of replacing the silver tube with a plastic one and should know how to care for the radiation reactions around the stoma.

TRACHEOSTOMY

This is an artificial opening into the trachea in the anterior aspect of the neck to allow breathing. A tube is inserted into the opening to keep it patent (Fig. 16.1, Fig. 16.2).

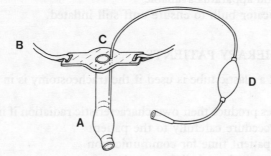

Fig. 16.1 Disposable, cuffed, tracheostomy tube
A — Inflatable cuff
B — Neck tapes
C — Opening
D — Indicating bulb, to check cuff inflated

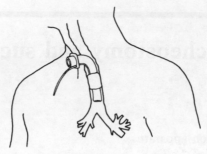

Fig. 16.2   Tracheostomy tube in position

Indications for performing a tracheostomy

Paralysis of the vocal cords/oedema of the vocal cords
Obstruction of the upper respiratory tract
To allow for maximum efficiency if a ventilator is used
Laryngeal tumour.

Patient care

Instil confidence as the patient will be apprehensive
Pencil and paper required for communication
Do not dislodge the tube
Do not remove or undo the tapes holding the tube in position
The patient should remain in the department for the minimum
length of time
Do not leave the patient unattended
Have suction apparatus available
Check indicator bulb to ensure cuff still inflated.

RADIOTHERAPY PATIENTS

Check that a plastic tube is used if the tracheostomy is in the treat-
ment field
(Silver tubes produce their own characteristic radiation if irradiated)
Explain procedure carefully to the patient
Allow the patient time for communication
Give patient an alarm bell for use during treatment
Show the patient that he can be seen by the radiographers
throughout the treatment
Special care should be given if the tracheostomy is recent

Keep suction apparatus close by

Check a power point is available

Stoma area should be kept free of mucus and debris

Gentle swabbing of the stoma area but vigorous washing is contraindicated.

SUCTION

Types of suction apparatus

Portable (Fig. 16.3) — involves the use of a foot pump and catheter

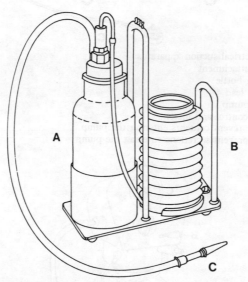

Fig. 16.3 Portable suction apparatus
A — Receiving bottle
B — Foot pump
C — Catheter attachment

Electrical (Fig. 16.4) — mounted on casters and is plugged into the wall

Pipeline (Fig. 16.5) — wall mounted with an independent vacuum and few controls

Use of suction

Explain the procedure to the patient

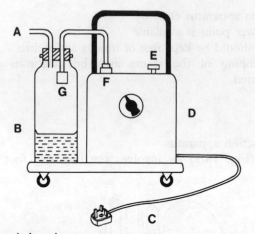

Fig. 16.4 Electrical suction apparatus
A — Catheter attachment
B — Receiving bottle
C — Electrical lead
D — Vacuum pump
E — Pressure control and meter
F — Filter to prevent contents entering the pump
G — Valve to prevent secretions entering the pump

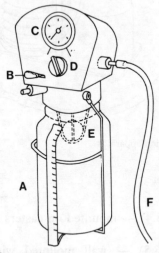

Fig. 16.5 Pipeline suction apparatus
A — Receiving bottle
B — On/off switch
C — Pressure gauge
D — Suction control
E — Float chamber
F — Tubing to catheter

Check that the apparatus is working correctly and leave switched on
Clear the airway, remove patient's false teeth
Place patient supine
Cover the chest with a protective sheet
Sterile procedure
Choose an appropriate catheter, preferably with staggered openings
Wash hands
Wearing disposable gloves, connect the catheter to the apparatus
Keep the catheter tip covered until required
Holding the catheter 10 cm from the end, place the catheter in the patient's mouth
Pass the catheter as far as is comfortable for the patient
Switch on the machine, occlude Y tube to create suction
Withdraw the catheter, slowly rotating it at the same time
Use the catheter once only
  NB. The catheter should remain in the trachea for a maximum of 10 seconds.

Suction for a patient who has had a tracheostomy

Sterile procedure
Patient's neck is extended
Select a catheter half the diameter of the tracheostomy tube, insert into trachea, pushing gently down to the carina — procedure as above.
  Throughout the procedure the colour of the patient is observed as oxygen may be required. At the end of the procedure the catheter is disposed of and the apparatus cleaned.

17. Fractures

INTRODUCTION

Radiographing bones for possible fractures may form a substantial part of a radiographer's work. They must be able to recognise the signs and symptoms associated with common fractures which could warn them of impending positioning difficulties.

A knowledge of the first aid treatment of fractures is necessary for patients admitted via the accident and emergency department.

For Therapy radiographers, the most common fractures encountered will be caused by malignant deposits in the bone which may completely destroy the bone tissue in one area.

For the care of lifting and moving these patients, see Chapter 5 on transportation of patients.

A fracture is a break in bone continuity.

TYPES OF FRACTURE

Simple/closed — Where there is no break in the skin surface
Compound/open — There is a loss of continuity of the skin surface and therefore a risk of infection
Complicated — There is associated injury with an organ or vessel
Transverse (Fig. 17.1) — A horizontal break.

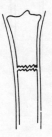

Fig. 17.1 Transverse fracture

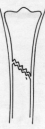

Fig. 17.2 Oblique fracture

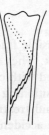

Fig. 17.3 Spiral fracture

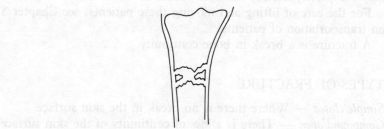

Fig. 17.4 Comminuted fracture

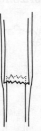

Fig. 17.5 Impacted fracture

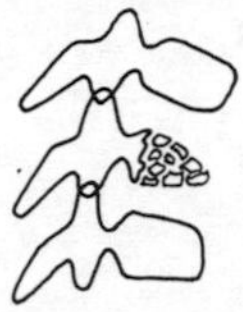

Fig. 17.6   Compression fracture

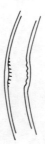

Fig. 17.7   Greenstick fracture

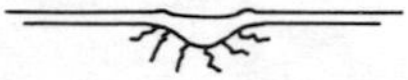

Fig. 17.8   Depressed fracture

Oblique (Fig. 17.2) An oblique break
Spiral (Fig. 17.3) Twists round, most common site is tibia
Comminuted (Fig. 17.4) Contains fragments of bone
Impacted (Fig. 17.5) The ends of the bones overlap
Compression (Fig. 17.6) The bone is crushed
Greenstick (Fig. 17.7) The bone appears bent — occurs in young children
Depressed (Fig. 17.8) Occurs when the bone (most commonly the skull) is struck by a hard object
Pathological Occurs because of underlying disease making the affected bone more susceptible to damage e.g. malignant tumour deposits.

Local signs and symptoms

Pain/swelling/bruising
Abnormal mobility
Deformity
Loss of use of limbs
Shortening — if occurring in a limb
Haemorrhage
Crepitus — not active sort.

Treatment of the fracture

Immobilise (temporary)
Reduce
Immobilise
Rehabilitate

Emergency treatment

Reassure the patient
Cover any wound with a clean cloth/arrest any haemorrhage
Immobilise with care (always supporting above and below the fracture site) by using —
   slings
   splints
   bandages
If possible, elevate a fractured limb
Treat patient for shock
Keep movement to a minimum
Nothing given by mouth

Reduction methods

Closed manipulation — a quick method usually performed under general anaesthetic, no surgery required.

Mechanical traction — a slow method, performed by attaching a weight to the lower limb which slowly pulls the leg, therefore opposing the muscular pull. Done to realign bones/joints, overcome muscle spasm, immobilise fractures/joints, correct deformity caused by shortened ligaments/tendons.

Open reduction — a quick method, performed in theatre.

Immobilisation

Plaster of Paris — must not be too tight. A note is made of any pain/swelling/discomfort.

Splints — can be made of aluminium with foam backing, plastic, polystyrene.

Rehabilitation

Restores normal function
Begins after reduction — the patient is encouraged to move fingers/toes.

COMMON FRACTURES

Bennett's — of first metacarpal, an oblique fracture/dislocation involving the first carpo-metacarpal joint
Colles' — fracture of the lower end of radius and ulna with backward displacement of the radius
Smith's — fracture of the lower end of radius and ulna with forward displacement of the radius
March — stress fracture of a metatarsal, often a hair-line crack
Pott's — fracture/fracture dislocation of the ankle
Supracondylar — lower end of humerus, elbow is displaced backwards.

Healing of fractures

A blood clot is formed due to damaged blood vessels
Within 24 hours the haematoma is converted into vascular tissue
After 7 days osteoblasts lay down cartilage and osteoid tissue, forming provisional callus
Provisional callus is converted to 'normal bone' containing Haversian systems
Bone is moulded by osteoclasts and osteoblasts to regain original shape.

Factors influencing healing

Healing may be delayed by one, or more than one, of the following factors:
    Age — usually the older the person the slower the rate of

healing, due to decreased blood supply and slower metabolism
Poor diet
Vitamin deficiency
Infection — more common with compound fractures
Malunion — due to poor reduction
Foreign bodies, bone fragments present
Poor immobilisation

18. Haemorrhage

INTRODUCTION

It is important that student radiographers learn the treatment for haemorrhage because of the possibility of encountering a patient in the department needing immediate attention for a bleeding wound.

Diagnostic radiographers in the accident and emergency department may have to radiograph patients with external bleeding but it should be stressed that a potentially more serious problem could arise if an internal haemorrhage goes unnoticed.

Radiotherapy radiographers often have to deal with patients who are suffering with haemorrhaging wounds due to tumour involvement and they are also required to assist during routine skin biopsies which frequently involve having to control a haemorrhaging wound.

Haemorrhage is the escape of blood from blood vessels, resulting from damage caused by injury or disease.

TYPES OF HAEMORRHAGE

Arterial

Blood is bright red
Spurts under pressure
Blood comes from the proximal side of the wound except where there is free anastomosis e.g. radial and ulnar arteries.

Venous

Blood is dark purple
'Wells' up in an even stream
Is distal to the wound except when varicosed

Capillary

Blood is bright red
Oozes from the wound
Rarely forms large blood loss.

CLASSIFICATION

Primary

Occurs at the time of injury

Reactionary

Occurs a few hours after injury and within 24 hours
Shock/drugs inhibit the blood flow

Secondary

Occurs about 10 days after injury
Is always due to sepsis.

External

The skin surface is damaged, bleeding occurs

Internal

Bleeding inside the body, often not seen externally.

SIGNS AND SYMPTOMS OF SEVERE HAEMORRHAGE

Rise in pulse rate
Drop in blood pressure
Pallor
Subnormal temperature
Restlessness
Rapid, sighing respiration
Skin cold, clammy
Faintness/fainting
Thirst
Dilated pupils

Pain — if bleeding into the peritoneal cavity
Nausea.

TREATMENT OF HAEMORRHAGE

Internal

Keep the patient warm
Lie the patient down, raise the legs, unless contraindicated
Assist if vomiting — save the vomit for inspection
Do not give the patient anything to eat or drink
Send for medical aid.

External

Same general treatment as above
In addition:
Apply digital pressure on the wound, unless a foreign body is
present
Cover the wound with a sterile pad
If bleeding continues, cover the first pad with a second
If possible raise the limb above the level of the head (unless
injury to head/neck/shoulder in which case lie the patient flat).

If a foreign body is suspected

Apply digital pressure to the nearest pressure point:
for arterial bleeding — proximal to the injury
for venous bleeding — distal to the injury
NB. A tourniquet must not be applied as this may damage nerves,
increase the blood supply and if not released may cause gangrene.

TERMS ASSOCIATED WITH HAEMORRHAGE

Haematemesis

Vomiting of blood as a result of bleeding from the upper
gastrointestinal tract e.g. from a gastric or duodenal ulcer. The
blood has the appearance of 'coffee grounds' when it has been in
the stomach for a long time.

Haematoma

A swelling composed of blood which can occur in any part of the body e.g. extradural — between the dura and the skull, subdural — between the dura and the arachnoid matter, intracerebral — within the brain.

Haematuria

Blood in the urine, can be the result of renal damage, tumour in the renal tract or an inflammatory disorder of the urinary bladder.

Haemoptysis

Coughing up of blood from the respiratory tract as a result of carcinoma of the bronchus, pulmonary tuberculosis, bronchiectasis. The blood is bright red in colour and frothy.

Haemorrhoids (piles)

Dilated veins round the anal area. Tend to be a cause of bleeding from the lower intestinal tract.

Haemothorax

Blood in the pleural cavity, associated with chest injuries e.g. fractured ribs.

Blood volume

The amount of blood circulating in the body. In adult male equal to 5.5 litres.

19. Sterile dressings

INTRODUCTION

Diagnostic and therapeutic radiographers come into contact with open and infected wounds.

Patients involved in road traffic accidents come to accident and emergency departments often requiring an X-ray examination, whilst many patients are seen in the radiotherapy department with open and infected wounds due to tumour involvement in the skin. Radiographers have to be able to set up a sterile dressings trolley or tray and apply sterile dressings in the absence of any nursing help.

This section aims at dealing with basic sterile dressing technique which should be correctly practised to prevent the spread of infection to other patients and staff and to try and keep a clean wound free from infection. Any infection in a wound will seriously delay the healing process.

Staphylococcus aureus is a common pathogen in hospitals (staff and patients). Virulent, antibiotic resistant bacteria such as MRSA — methicillin resistant Staphylococcus aureus — has resulted in intensive infection control policies being implemented.

DRESSINGS

Required to protect broken skin from infection.

General principles

Dressings are only carried out if necessary
All instruments and dressings must be sterile
Air disturbance must be reduced to a minimum
The wound must be exposed for the minimum amount of time.

DRESSING TROLLEY

Ideally, trolley settings should be done in a room reserved only for this purpose.

The trolley should be cleaned with an antiseptic solution and dried.

Top shelf (sterile items)

A sterile CSSD pack is placed on the top shelf, containing:
Gauze swabs
Cotton wool balls
Sterile towels or paper drapes
Gallipots
Sterile dressings
4 pairs of dressing forceps

Bottom shelf (nonsterile items)

Bottle of cleansing lotion e.g. cetrimide 1%
Adhesive tape
Disposable bag for dirty dressings

MASKS

Usually worn to filter micro-organisms from the expired air and therefore prevent infection by the airborne route.

Precautions

Paper masks are worn for a maximum of 10 minutes (unless they become moist, when they should be discarded)
Mask must cover the nose and mouth
The tapes only should be handled when removing the mask
Once removed the mask should be discarded — not reworn.

BASIC DRESSING PROCEDURE (no touch technique)

Prepare trolley
Explain the procedure to the patient
Wash hands
Open pack (handling outside only)

Pour cleansing lotion into the gallipot (not holding the bottle over the sterile area)

Remove existing dressing with forceps and dispose of dressing

Wash hands

Clean the wound — each swab only used once
                                 clean from the inside to the outside
                                 dry the area

Cover with clean dressing using sterile forceps

Attach dressing with adhesive tape or bandages

Return unused instruments and dressings to CSSD for resterilisation.

Put dirty dressings into a clinical waste bag (follow waste disposal procedures).

20. Diabetes

INTRODUCTION

Patients attending the imaging or radiotherapy departments needing regular and controlled units of insulin to keep their diabetes under control require special consideration.

It could happen that a patient accidentally forgets to administer his insulin prior to attending the hospital or misses a meal because of a delay when he arrives at the hospital. Radiographers are expected to recognise the signs and symptoms of a diabetic or insulin coma and initiate the first aid treatment if necessary.

Patients attending the department on a regular basis should, if possible, be given an appointment time which does not disrupt their own routine.

As diabetes insipidus is a completely separate disease it is necessary to be able to distinguish between the two.

DIABETES MELLITUS

Beta cells of the pancreas in the Islets of Langerhans secrete insulin which plays a part in carbohydrate metabolism. If there is a deficiency in the amount of insulin produced diabetes mellitus results.

Normal serum glucose level = 4.5–6.9 mmol/l.

Diagnosis

Hyperglycaemia — excessive glucose in the blood
Glycosuria — glucose in the urine

Signs and symptoms

Thirst
Polyuria — excess urine production (contains sugar)

169

Weight loss (general emaciation)
Raised blood glucose.

Chronic complications

Decreased arterial function (poor circulation).

Diabetic coma (hyperglycaemic coma)

Occurs if the disease is untreated or if insulin had been omitted.

Signs

Slow onset, may be over days
Drowsiness/unconsciousness
Deep sighing breaths
Dry skin/flushed face
Smell of acetone on the breath
Fast thready pulse
Abdominal pain
Polyuria
Low blood pressure.

Treatment

Insulin is given

Insulin coma (hypoglycaemic coma)

Caused by an overdose of insulin, or lack of food at the appropriate time.

Signs and symptoms

Onset tends to be rapid
Sinking feeling and hunger
May tremble, appear drunk/confused/aggressive
Shallow or normal breathing
Sweating, moist, clammy skin
No breath odour
Faintness/unconsciousness
Fast pounding pulse
Blurred or double vision.

Treatment

Give sugar orally or, if unconscious, place in recovery position. An intravenous injection of glucose is given by a Medical Officer.

DIABETES INSIPIDUS (rare)

Occurs if the production of antidiuretic hormone, which is stored in the neurohypophysis (posterior lobe) of the pituitary gland, decreases.

Symptoms

Severe thirst
Passage of excessive amounts of dilute urine
Weakness
General emaciation.

THE DIABETIC PATIENT IN THE IMAGING DEPARTMENT

No special care required unless:
Starvation required e.g. if general anaesthetic is required, barium meal examinations
Diet modification e.g. abdominal preparation
If an ambulance is required, inform the ambulance centre of the patient's condition

Starvation

Patient asked: to omit insulin, to bring food and insulin with them
Placed first on the list and told how long the examination will be
Radiologist informed.

Diet modification

Only after consultation with a radiologist or the patient's general practitioner.

THE DIABETIC PATIENT IN THE RADIOTHERAPY DEPARTMENT

Appointment given to suit the patient (not at their mealtimes)
Ambulance service should be notified if a diabetic patient is using the transport services

Diabetic patients have an increased susceptibility to infection which must be borne in mind with radiotherapy patients
Often these patients suffer with circulatory problems and severe arteriosclerosis. They should not be placed in cold and draughty areas (no patient should be!)
Problems can arise if the insulin balance is upset due to patients becoming anorexic from the radiotherapy treatment.

21. Colostomy and ileostomy

INTRODUCTION

Radiographers in the imaging and radiotherapy department will have to deal with patients with a colostomy or ileostomy. These patients may be apprehensive of revealing their stoma to the radiographers and therefore they must receive reassurance from the radiographers that their problems will be understood and overcome.

Radiographers should know how to assist a patient with the removal of the drainage bag and be able to give advice on general management of the stoma following an X-ray examination or radiotherapy treatment, and should discuss any side effects resulting from the investigation or treatment.

COLOSTOMY/ILEOSTOMY

When a portion of either the colon (colostomy) or ileum (ileostomy) opens onto the anterior abdominal wall to form either a temporary or a permanent artificial anus (stoma) through which faeces are discharged.

Indications

Rest a diseased bowel e.g. Crohn's disease
Imperforate anus
Prior to surgery or after resection of diseased bowel e.g.
    Ulcerative colitis
    Diverticulosis
    Malignant tumour.

Diet

Patients should avoid constipation or diarrhoea
Food causing flatus or odour should be avoided.

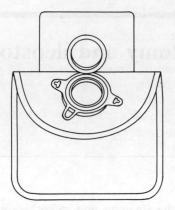

Fig. 21.1   Nondrainable stoma bag

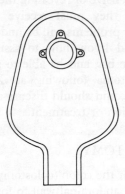

Fig. 21.2   Drainable stoma bag

Personal hygiene

Use of disposable colostomy bags (Fig. 21.1, Fig. 21.2)
Careful washing of the stoma
Use of self adhesive bags — prevent sore skin due to the indirect skin contact (see Fig. 21.1)
Patient/staff wash hands before and after handling the bags

Ileal conduit

The ureters are attached to the ileum, part of which forms a reservoir for urine. The urine drains to the anterior abdominal wall via the ileum.

Barium enema examination

Ensure clean colostomy bag available
Enema usually performed via the stoma
Careful catheterisation of the bowel through the stoma
May require a more dilute solution
Care not to overfill bowel.
Ensure facilities available for the patient with regard to hand washing, changing and the correct disposal of the bag.

CARE OF THE PATIENT IN THE RADIOTHERAPY DEPARTMENT

Pelvic or abdominal irradiation may follow surgical treatment for carcinoma of the rectum if residual disease is present
The area of the stoma is kept out of the treatment area unless there is known disease present
Following radiotherapy, diarrhoea may be a problem
Attention to diet — no foods which could enhance the problem of diarrhoea
If any anti-diarrhoea drug is prescribed, care must be taken to prevent constipation
High fluid intake must be emphasised
Anti-emetics required for nausea or vomiting.

22. Nursing procedures

INTRODUCTION

The general principles of nursing procedures should be taught to all hospital personnel who come into contact with patients.

Radiographing or treating hospitalised patients is only one part of the nursing programme for the patient. It is important that the care of the patient does not become isolated within individual departments of a hospital. An understanding of general nursing procedures by student radiographers will help the integration of the total nursing care for the patients.

Practical experience of these procedures should be gained on selected wards soon after the commencement of training.

BEDMAKING

Principles

To enhance patient comfort
To ensure the economical use of equipment.

Articles required

Receptacles for soiled linen
Linen
    bottom sheet
    waterproof sheet
    draw sheet
    top sheet
    pillow cases
    blankets

Procedure

Clear patient's locker top
Pull out the racks on the end of the bed
Loosen the sheets
Remove blankets
Change the sheets
Dispose of the dirty linen
Replace the blankets
Reposition the rack
Replace articles on the locker.

Patient considerations

Patient's face should never be covered by linen
Clothes should never be drawn tightly over the body

Bed accessories

Bed tables
Bed cradles — relieve pressure/weight of sheets over injured parts of the body.
Bed elevators — used to raise either end of the bed e.g. to aid breathing or as a treatment for shock.
Rings/airbeds/cushions — to reduce pressure and therefore prevent decubitus ulcers (pressure sores).
Ripple beds — alternate sections fill and then empty, used to prevent decubitus ulcers.
Pulleys — enable patients on traction to lift themselves up to give themselves exercise, and makes bedmaking easier.

Continental quilts

These have now replaced 'normal' bedding in some hospitals.

Advantages

More comfortable for the patient
Create less dust therefore more hygienic
Allow easy access for nursing care
Light in weight
Easy to clean

Saves bedmaking time
Helps create a better atmosphere for long-term residents.

Disadvantages

Some are not constructed of flame retardant material and are therefore thought to be a fire risk.

Position in bed

Supine — for relaxation, contraindications —
  Patients who are elderly
  Patients who have had abdominal surgery
  Patients who are chronically ill
Prone — for spinal injuries
Semi-recumbent — for medical and surgical patients
Erect, sitting — for convalescent patients
Coma position — for unconscious patients.

Dangers of bed rest

  Deep vein thrombosis — changes in walls of veins causing clots, stasis of blood in the vein
  Pneumonia — inflammation of lung tissue
  Urinary complications — retention, infection, bedwetting
  Decubitus ulcers (pressure sores) — areas of inflammation caused by prolonged pressure occurring usually on elbows, buttocks and heels

PRESSURE AREA CARE

Causes of decubitus ulcers

External

Friction   — patient being dragged over uneven surfaces
Shearing   — blood vessels are torn, can occur if the patient is
                   scratched
Pressure   — from bony areas and contact with wet or damp
                   surfaces and hard objects e.g. crumbs, cassettes.

Internal

Old age
General health of patient
Immobility of patient
Diminished ability to appreciate pain
Pathological conditions — diabetes mellitus, general paralysis.

Prevention of decubitus ulcers

Patient moved 2 hourly
Reduce pressure e.g. by using a ripple bed
Well balanced diet — high protein content
Prevent patient becoming anaemic

Treatment of pressure areas

Patient is moved 2 hourly
Use of silicone cream — protects from moisture
Use of ripple beds, water immersion beds, air rings, sheepskins
If an ulcer develops it is treated with aseptic precautions to prevent
infection
   NB. Massaging of the skin is now contraindicated as it is a form
of friction and is therefore thought to encourage decubitus ulcers.

Norton score

A method used for assessing the risk to a patient of developing a
decubitus ulcer. If the final score is under 14 the patient is at risk.

BED BATHS

Articles required

Jug of hot water
Basin
Soap
Talcum powder
Beaker, toothbrush, toothpaste, receiver
Hairbrush and comb
Nail scissors
Face and hand towels
Bath towels
Clean linen for the patient and the bed.

Patient preparation

Inform patient of procedure
Draw bed curtains
Offer bedpan/urinal
Close windows
Remove top bedclothes
Place towels over and under the patient
Remove patient's clothing.

Method

Wash and dry
  face, neck, ears,
  chest, arms.
change the water
  lower chest, abdomen
  lower limbs
  back
  genital region — washed by patient if possible
Talcum powder is applied

Additional care

Nails cut if required
Hair washed if necessary
Teeth cleaned

After-care

Patient dresses in clean clothes
Bed is remade
Drink is given
Windows are opened
Curtains drawn back.

MOUTH CARE

Complications of mouth neglect

Crustations on lips and teeth
Cracked lips
Furring of the tongue

Herpes — mouth sores
Odious taste
Can destroy sense of taste
Halitosis — bad breath.

Can lead to infection of

Stomach	— gastritis
Lungs	— inhalation pneumonia
Middle ear	— otitis media
Parotid gland	— parotitis
Tonsils	— tonsillitis
Tongue	— glossitis.

Cleansing by the patient

Clean the teeth
Clean dentures with warm water and cleansing powder
Mouthwash given.

To cleanse a patient's mouth

Remove dentures
Clean the dentures with a brush
Swab mouth with liquid, using a swab and forceps
Clean teeth from gum to crown
Give a mouthwash
Return dentures
Wipe mouth dry.

VOMITING

Causes

Stomach irritants
Stomach disease
Chemotherapy
Pregnancy
Infection
Raised intracranial pressure.

Complications which may occur

Dehydration
Alkalosis
Ketosis
Sodium loss.

Patient care

Reassure the patient
Provide vomit bowel and tissues
Support patient if required
Provide a mouthwash
Wipe mouth dry
Retain vomit for inspection
Lie patient on his/her side and give privacy
Medical Officer asked to see patient.

BEDPANS AND URINALS

Giving a bedpan

Place screens round the patient
Ensure the bedpan is warm and dry
Take the pan to the patient
Lift the patient if necessary
Adjust and support the patient if necessary
If possible, leave the patient alone
Cleanse the patient, using toilet tissue or swabs
Provide hand washing facilities.

Emptying the bedpan

Inspect the contents for blood, unusual colour
Flush the pan
Inspect to see if clean
Sterilise if necessary
Wash hands.

Disposable bedpans

Strengthened cardboard (papier-mâché)
Support for the bedpan is required — in the form of a metal frame

After use inspect contents
Dispose of pan and contents.

Urinals

Take the urinal to the patient covered
Assist if necessary
Check contents for blood etc.
Record the volume of urine if necessary
Disinfect or sterilise the urinal
Place the urinal upside down to drain
Wash hands.

LUMBAR PUNCTURE

Insertion of a needle into lumbar subarachnoid space to gain access to cerebrospinal fluid.

Indications

To remove cerebrospinal fluid for analysis
To measure the pressure of cerebrospinal fluid
To introduce a contrast agent to examine the nerve roots and spinal canal
To introduce cytotoxic drugs.

Equipment — sterile procedure

Swabs/skin cleanser
Syringe
Needles and stilette
Local anaesthetic
Lumbar puncture needle
Manometer
Sterile specimen bottles
Contrast agent/cytotoxic agent
Sterile towels.

Procedure

Explanation to patient
Patient lies on his side

Hips and knees flexed to separate vertebral processes
Skin cleaned
Local anaesthetic introduced over the site of the puncture
Lumbar puncture needle introduced between 2nd and 3rd lumbar
vertebra, (below termination of the spinal cord) into subarachnoid
space
Stilette removed

Investigations

> *Pressure* — taken with a manometer attached to the needle
> (normal 75—150 mm)
> *Sample* — a small quantity of cerebrospinal fluid is collected
> in the specimen bottle and is sent for analysis
> *Radiography* — contrast agent is introduced during radiculo-
> graphy

After-care

Needle withdrawn
Sterile dressing applied.

23. Temperature, pulse, respiration and blood pressure

INTRODUCTION

When dealing with physically sick patients it is often necessary to carry out an accurate assessment of a patient's physical condition. An indication of how ill a patient is can be found by taking a patient's temperature, pulse and respiration. The radiographer is often the person having the immediate contact with the patient which means she is the person who has to make the preliminary assessment of that patient.

Student radiographers should gain practical experience in these skills on the ward and in the department.

TEMPERATURE

Features of a typical clinical thermometer (Fig. 23.1)

10 cm long graduated glass tube with a 'bulb' at one end
A magnifying lens on one side

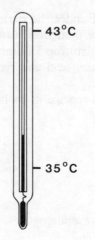

Fig. 23.1 Clinical thermometer

A short temperature range, usually 35°C–43°C
Mercury filled bulb and central column
Can be sterilised using chemical solutions
Unfortunately is breakable
Constriction above the bulb to retain the position of the mercury
Self registering
Accurate if used correctly
  NB. A rectal thermometer has a wider, alcohol filled, bulb which
is either blue, or has a blue dot to identify it.

General principles

Temperature should not be taken directly after:
  a hot bath
  a hot drink
  smoking.
Temperature may be taken:
  orally
  rectally
  in axilla/groin.
Patient has his own thermometer which is wiped with swabs before
use. An explanation is given to the patient regarding the procedure.

Orally

Method

Thermometer is shaken to read below 35.5°C by 'flicking' the
thermometer
Thermometer is placed under the patient's tongue
Patient is asked to close their lips but not bite
Thermometer is left in situ for 5 minutes
Remove the thermometer, read and record immediately
Shake mercury down
Wipe thermometer and replace in its holder.

Contraindications

Infants
Unconscious patients
Delirious patients
Insane patients
Patients who suffer from epilepsy

If mouth closure is inconvenient — e.g. cough,
obstructed nasal breathing
dyspnoea (difficult breathing)

Rectally

(The normal reading is 2° higher than skin temperature and 1°
higher than oral temperature).
The thermometer has a wider bulb which is coloured and filled
with alcohol.

Method

Thermometer is shaken to read below 35°C
The bulb is lubricated
Patient lies on their side
Thermometer is inserted 5 cm into the rectum
Thermometer is left in situ for 5 minutes
Read and record immediately
Clean the thermometer.

Axilla/groin

The normal reading is 1° less than oral and 2° less than rectal
temperature.

Method

The skin surfaces must be dry
The thermometer is shaken to read below 35°C
The thermometer is placed under the axilla or in the groin
Skin surfaces are pressed together to exclude air
Thermometer is left in situ for 5 minutes
Read and record immediately
Clean the thermometer.

Digital thermometers

Used for oral, arm and skin temperatures
Rectal probes are available
Overall range 20–50°C
10–20 seconds response time
Temperature on a digital display

Display can be 'held' for reference purposes
Battery operated.

Electronic thermometers (Fig. 23.2)

Similar to digital but with a meter display
Disposable probe covers are available
5 second response time
If probe covers used, 9–12 seconds response time
Probe sterilised with alcohol
Battery operated.

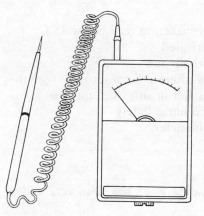

Fig. 23.2 Electronic thermometer

Recording the temperature

The temperature is recorded on the patient's chart (Fig. 23.3) with a dot which is joined to the previous dot with either a straight line if it is above or below the previous reading, or a loop if the previous

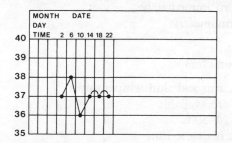

Fig. 23.3 Temperature chart

reading is the same. The thermometer should always be read in good light and recording must be done immediately.

PULSE

Each pulse represents a cardiac cycle and can be felt where an artery passes superficially and lies over a bone i.e. at a pressure point.

Common sites

Radial pulse — wrist (palmer aspect of the lateral side)
Femoral pulse — groin
Carotid pulse — neck.

Checking the pulse rate (radial)

Explain the procedure to the patient
Ensure the patient is at rest
The hand and arm should be supported
Place your fingers (not the thumb as there is a pulse in the thumb) over the pulse to be recorded
If regular, count the beats for 30 seconds
Double the number and record immediately
If irregular, the beats are counted for a full minute.

Electronic pulse monitor (Fig. 23.4)

A spring-loaded photocell is clipped on the finger
A diode lamp flashes with the pulse rate
Scale measurement range 30–200 beats/minute
10 second response time
Battery operated.

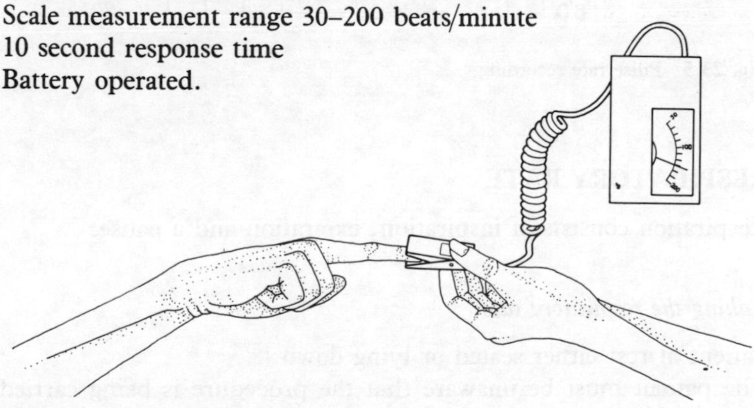

Fig. 23.4 Electronic pulse monitor

In addition to the rate, note the

Tension — bounding/thready
Rhythm — regular/irregular
Volume — full/normal/small.

In a normal pulse the

Rate — corresponds to the age of the patient
Rhythm — regular
Volume — moderate
Tension — not easily compressed.

Recording the pulse rate

The pulse is recorded immediately on the patient's chart (Fig. 23.5) with a dot which is joined to the previous dot with either a straight line if it is above or below the previous reading, or a loop if the previous reading is the same.

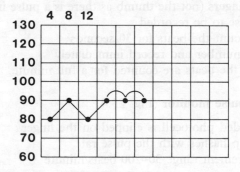

Fig. 23.5 Pulse rate recording

RESPIRATORY RATE

Respiration consists of inspiration, expiration and a pause.

Taking the respiratory rate

Patient at rest either seated or lying down
The patient must be unaware that the procedure is being carried out

One rise and fall of the chest equals one respiration
It is usual to count the rate whilst appearing to take the pulse
The rate is counted for 30 seconds and then doubled
If irregular, the rate is counted for a full minute
Record immediately.

In addition to the rate, note the

Depth of respiration
Regularity
Rhythm
Sound.

Recording the respiratory rate

The respiratory rate is recorded immediately on the patient's chart
(Fig. 23.6) with a dot which is joined to the previous dot with either
a straight line if it is above or below the previous reading, or a loop
if the previous reading is the same.

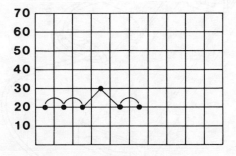

Fig. 23.6   Respiratory rate recording

BLOOD PRESSURE

Factors maintaining blood pressure:
   Pumping force of the heart — cardiac output
   Quantity of blood in the body and the blood volume
   Elasticity of the blood vessels
   Resistance to the passage of blood in the vessels — peripheral
   resistance
   Viscosity of the blood.

Manual sphygmomanometer (Fig. 23.7)

Instrument used indirectly to measure blood pressure which consists of a:

Mercury manometer in millimetres
Collapsible arm band
Pump and valve

Also required is a stethoscope.

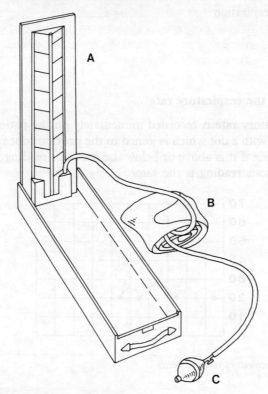

Fig. 23.7 Manual sphygmomanometer
A — Graduated mercury column
B — Inflatable arm band
C — Hand pump

Method of taking blood pressure

Patient should be at rest
Patient extends their arm and it is supported
Arm band is placed round the patient's arm, above the elbow

Arm band is inflated
The radial pulse is palpated during inflation
Remember the level of mercury when the pulse disappears
The arm band is inflated for a further 5 millimetres
Place the stethoscope below the crease of the elbow
Release the air from the arm band until the first sound is heard
The level of mercury gives the systolic pressure (when the heart is contracting and blood is forced through the arteries).
Listen until the sound reaches the maximum
1 soft sound followed by a second soft sound is then heard
The level of mercury gives the diastolic pressure (when the chambers of the heart are full of blood).
Arm band deflated.

Electronic sphygmomanometer (Fig. 23.8)

No stethoscope required
Cuff placed round the arm, 4–5 cm above the antecubital fossa
Cuff inflated by repeatedly squeezing the bulb
Cuff automatically deflates and manometer needle drops
First flash/bleep denotes systolic pressure
Unit continues to flash and bleep with the blood pressure sounds
Last flash/bleep indicates the diastolic pressure
Battery powered
Dial range 20–200 mm of mercury (mm Hg).

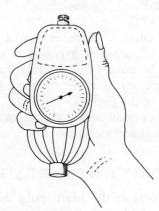

Fig. 23.8   Electronic sphygmomanometer

Recording the blood pressure

The blood pressure is recorded immediately on the patient's chart

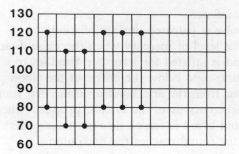

Fig. 23.9 Blood pressure recording

(Fig 23.9), usually at right angles to the other readings. A straight line joins the diastolic and the systolic pressures.

TERMS ASSOCIATED WITH TEMPERATURE

Fever: Pyrexia 37.2°C–40.5°C.

Hyperpyrexia: A dangerous condition with high body temperature above 40.5°C.

Hypothermia: General lowering of body temperature, may occur when heat loss exceeds heat production. Results following shock or injury, fatal if uncontrolled. Temperatures are usually below 35°C and therefore a special thermometer 24°C–41°C is required.

Normal: 35.5°C–37.2°.

Subnormal: Below 35°C.

Pel-Ebstein fever: Often a characteristic of Hodgkin and non Hodgkin lymphoma. Consists of a period of pyrexia — often as high as 40°C lasting between 3 and 10 days, followed by a period of normal temperature lasting about the same length of time, followed by the return of the pyrexia.

Pyrexia: Elevation of body temperature above normal.

PUO: Pyrexia of unknown origin.

TERMS ASSOCIATED WITH PULSE RATE

Bradycardia: Slowness of the heart, pulse less than 60/minute, can occur during sleep/old age/hypothermia, or as a result of treatment by certain drugs.

Normal: Adults — 65 to 80 beats/minute (women 5 beats faster than men)

New-born infant — 120 to 140 beats/minute

Child age 5 — 100 beats/minute
Old age — pulse slows
Very old age — pulse quickens

Tachycardia: Increase in heart beat above normal limits, pulse rate 160–200 beats/minute occurs following shock/haemorrhage/ heart condition/hyperthermia/action of certain drugs.

Sinus arrhythmia: Heart rate increases on inspiration and decreases on expiration. Found in healthy adults.

TERMS ASSOCIATED WITH RESPIRATION

Apnoea: Associated with dyspnoea, absence of breathing for short periods.

Asthma: Gasping for breath due to spasm of the muscle walls of the bronchi.

Bronchiectasis: Abnormally dilated bronchi in the lungs, patient therefore prone to bronchial obstruction.

Cheyne-Stokes respiration: A cyclic pattern of irregular breathing occurring in patients with cerebral disease especially where there is raised intracranial pressure. Slow and shallow to start, progressing in speed and depth to a maximum then depressed again. Finally there is a period of apnoea for about 15 seconds and the cycle begins again.

Dyspnoea: Difficulty in breathing e.g. obstruction of airway, can be caused by heart disease. Patients are nursed semi-recumbent.

Haemoptysis: Coughing up of blood from the respiratory tract.

Normal respiration rate: 16–20 breaths/minute.

Sighing: Long slow inspiration followed by rapid expiration.

Stertorous: Breathing noisy, cheeks puffed in and out with each breath.

Wheezing: Rattling noises occur when air is forced through fluid.

TERMS ASSOCIATED WITH BLOOD PRESSURE

CCF: Congestive cardiac failure.

Hypertension: High blood pressure (can be due to renal disease) caused by narrowing of arteries causing resistance to peripheral circulation.

Hypotension: Low blood pressure.

Normal blood pressure: $\dfrac{120}{80}$ $\dfrac{\text{Systolic}}{\text{Diastolic}}$

Infancy: 50 (Diastolic) 70–90 (Systolic)

Childhood: 60 (Diastolic) 80–100 (Systolic)
Adolescence: 60 (Diastolic) 90–110 (Systolic)
Young adult: 60–70 (Diastolic) 110–125 (Systolic)
Adult: 80–90 (Diastolic) 130–150 (Systolic).

24. Catheterisation and intubation

INTRODUCTION

Although it is unlikely that a student radiographer will have to catheterise a patient there will be occasions when they will have to radiograph or treat patients with catheters in situ.

During certain diagnostic examinations the student may have to assist in the catheterisation of patients and it is therefore important that they understand the principles of catheterisation.

A chart outlining some of the more common catheters is available for reference purposes.

CATHETERISATION

The introduction of a tube into the body for the purpose of:
Discharging the fluid contents of a cavity
Establishing the patency of a canal
Introducing an agent into a cavity.

INTUBATION

The introduction of a tube into a hollow organ to keep it open e.g. into the larynx to ensure the passage of air, in general anaesthesia.

Introduction of a catheter

Catheterisation of the bladder is a sterile procedure and care must be taken:
Not to introduce micro-organisms
Not to damage the urethra.

Indications

Relieve urinary retention
Prevent bladder distension
Incontinence
Unconscious patients may require catheterisation.

Female patients

Urethral opening is swabbed
Using sterile gloves, or forceps, the catheter is introduced about
5 cm into the urethra
The catheter is attached to the patient's thigh, to prevent it from
becoming dislodged.

Male patients

The urethral opening is cleaned
The urethra is anaesthetised (lignocaine gel).

After 5 minutes

The catheter is introduced using an aseptic technique
The catheter is attached to the patient's thigh.

If the catheter becomes displaced

Do not reinsert as this will contaminate the bladder
Report the occurrence.

If the catheter comes out

Do not reinsert
Report the occurrence.

Disposable catheters

Advantages

Hygenic
Time saving
Readily available
Conveniently disposed of.

Disadvantages

Large supplies are required
Disposal must be efficient
Cannot be tested prior to use.

Foley catheters (Fig. 24.1)

Can be used on radiotherapy wards for patients with dysuria
Patients with carcinoma of the bladder are catheterised prior to performing a localising cystogram.

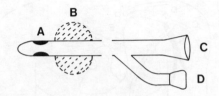

Fig. 24.1 Foley catheter
A — Eyelet for drainage
B — Inflatable balloon filled with sterile water
C — For urinary bag attachment
D — Side tube for inflating the balloon

If difficulties are expected during the treatment e.g. dysuria, then the catheter may be left in place until the patient is able to pass urine easily.

Principle of catheter insertion is the same as before, but the balloon, found at the proximal end of the catheter, is inflated with sterile water or air which keeps the catheter in place.

CENTRAL VENOUS CATHETERISATION

Catheterisation via the venous system into superior or inferior vena cava.

Uses

Monitoring central venous pressure
Total parenteral nutrition
Long-term/frequent administration of drugs — chemotherapy drugs, antibiotics, transfusion products
Taking blood samples.

Procedure

A central venous catheter commonly used is the Hickman.
Silicone rubber catheter which can be tunnelled under the skin into
e.g. right subclavian vein
Passes into right atrium of the heart
Allows patients with malignant disease to receive intravenous
chemotherapy and support treatment without repeated venepuncture through the skin

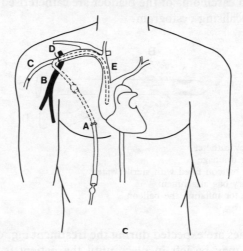

Fig. 24.2 Position of the Hickman line
A — Dacron cuff at exit site of Hickman line
B — Axillary vein
C — Cephalic vein
D — Incision
E — Superior vena cava

Distal end fitted with Luer-lok injectable cap
Strict aseptic conditions for handling catheter
Catheter kept patent by flushing heparin though.

TYPES OF CATHETERS/TUBES

Name	Material	Use	Sterilisation method
Drainage tubes	Rubber	Draining body cavities	Autoclaving
Foley catheter	Silicone	Bladder intubation (self retaining)	Autoclaving
Franklin catheter	Soft rubber	Rectal intubation	Autoclaving
Jaques'	Soft rubber	Rectal intubation	Autoclaving
Jaques' (disposable)	Polythene	Bladder intubation	Gamma radiation
Kifa (disposable)	Polythene	Aortography	Gamma radiation
Magill's laryngeal and bronchial tubes	Polythene	Bronchography Resuscitation	Gamma radiation
Nasal catheter	Rubber	Bronchography Oxygen administration	Autoclaving
Oesophageal tube (disposable)	Polythene	Gastric feeds Duodenal/small bowel intubation	Gamma radiation
Rectal catheter	Soft rubber	Rectal intubation	Autoclaving
Ryle's tube (disposable)	Polythene	Duodenal/small bowel intubation	Gamma radiation
Tiemann's catheter	Soft rubber	Male bladder catheterisation	Autoclaving
Ureteric catheter	Polythene	Retrograde urogram	Gamma radiation

25. Fire procedure

INTRODUCTION

Whatever the nature of employment in the Health Service it is directed to the support and protection of the existence and well being of human life. A knowledge of how to prevent fire and what action to take in the event of fire is very necessary for all hospital staff. Staff are required to attend lectures and fire drills.

This section on fire safety is therefore intended to be complementary to training which is received in the hospital. The traditional approach to fire protection is to identify and seek to eliminate the causes of fire, or failing that, to detect a fire as early as possible and contain it whilst it is being extinguished.

MAJOR CAUSES OF FIRE IN A DEPARTMENT

Misuse of electricity
Sunshine and matches
Faults in heating systems
Spontaneous combustion
Improper refuse disposal
Inflammable gases.

The major hazard for radiographers is the electrical fire. With few exceptions, fires of electrical origin occur due to lack of reasonable care in the use or maintenance of electrical installations and apparatus. The power used in radiographic equipment is capable of igniting insulation or other combustibles if the equipment is not adequate to carry the load or is not properly used, installed and maintained.

Common causes of electrical fires

Failure of insulation giving rise to short circuits or earth faults

Overheating of cables or equipment
Ignition of flammable substances by electrostatic discharge
    The second major hazard is film storage, although X-ray film is classed as non-flammable it has a combustibility similar to that of paper with the additional danger of dense volumes of carbon monoxide and other toxic gases.

FIRE PREVENTION

Be familiar with the local fire procedure
Know your emergency number
Ensure fire doors are not obstructed
Know the position of:
    Fire alarms
    Nearest fire appliances and how to operate them
    Fire assembly points
    First aid and resuscitation equipment.

Fire equipment should be checked on a regular basis. It is usual for the date of the last check to be written on the appliance.

Types of appliance available

The following is the British Standard colour coding for appliances:
Black extinguisher — carbon dioxide
    electrical fires
Red extinguisher   — water
    fires involving free-burning carbonaceous material
Blue extinguisher   — dry powder
    all types of fire
Hose   — water
    fires involving free-burning material
Fire blanket
    smothers person with burning clothes
    fires involving fat or oil.

It is important always to read the information on the body of the extinguisher in order to check the type and the operating instructions.

FIRE ROUTINE

Keep calm and reassure patients

Break glass on fire alarm/dial emergency number
Remove patients from the room but consider your own safety
Switch off the mains supply/remove combustible gases, if possible
For imaging equipment, use a black fire extinguisher, aiming at the base of the fire but only if no personal risk of danger
   NB. Try to avoid inhalation of the vapour, as carbon dioxide is an asphyxiant.
If smoke present — keep low
When leaving the room ensure that the doors and windows are closed
Do not re-enter the room.

Operation of equipment

Black, carbon dioxide cylinder

Hold neck (not the horn)
Remove the pin
Direct the nozzle at the fire
Firmly squeeze the handle.

Red, water cylinder

Place cylinder on the floor 4 metres from the fire
Kneel beside the cylinder
Hold the nozzle firmly
Remove the safety device
Strike (do not press) the knob
Aim at the base of the fire.

Hose

Turn on at the wall
Take to the fire (4 metres distant)
Turn on
Aim at the base of the fire.

Fire blanket

Hold blanket so that your hands and body are protected
Gently place over the fire
Leave in place until cool

Remember

Fire is an alarming threat in any situation. In a hospital where the safety and lives of colleagues and often helpless patients are at stake, it can be terrifying and tragic. The dangers and ill effects of smoke cannot be over-emphasised. Prevention is the first and best precaution, be constantly alert for fire risks of any kind.

Glossary

Abscess   a cavity which contains pus
Aerobe   micro-organism which requires oxygen to live e.g. surface wounds
Aetiology   study of causes of disease
Albuminuria   abnormal amount of albumin in the urine
Allergy   reaction to a substance e.g. iodine
Alzheimer's disease   presenile dementia
Ambulant   walking
Amenorrhoea   lack of menstruation
Amniocentesis   removal of amniotic fluid to estimate alpha protein level
Amnesia   loss of memory
Ampoule   container, usually glass, for sterile solutions
Anaerobe   micro-organism which does not need oxygen to live e.g. gangrene
Anaesthetic   drug producing loss of feeling
Analgesic   drug which relieves pain
Anaphylaxis   hypersensitivity/allergic reaction
Aneurysm   abnormal dilation of an artery
Anorexia   loss of appetite
Antibiotic   substance used to fight against infection
Antibody   substance either natural or introduced that helps protect the body from infection
Antiemetic   agent which prevents nausea and vomiting
Antigen   substance that stimulates the production of antibodies
Antihistamine   substance introduced to counteract an allergy
Antiseptic   agent that stops or inhibits the growth of bacteria but does not necessarily kill them
Anuria   arrest of urinary output
Aperient   mild drug given to produce peristaltic action and therefore bowel emptying

Apnoea   cessation of breathing
Arterial haemorrhage   bleeding from an artery
Arterio-venous shunt   direct connection between an artery and a vein
Arthritis   inflammation of a joint
Arthrodesis   fusion of a joint, usually by surgical means
Arthroplasty   surgical formation of a joint
Ascites   accumulation of serous fluid in the peritoneal cavity
Asepsis   exclusion of micro-organisms
Asphyxia   unconsciousness resulting from lack of oxygen
Ataxia   lack of voluntary muscular co-ordination
Atheroma   fatty degeneration of an artery wall
Atresia   closure of normal opening or canal e.g. oesophageal atresia in infants
Autoclave   equipment for sterilising articles e.g. by using steam under pressure
Autoimmunity   production of antibodies against subject's own tissue
Bacteria   infective micro-organism
Barrier nursing   method of nursing an infectious patient
Bedpan   a portable receptacle for receiving urine and faeces
Biopsy   removal of tissue from the living to determine the histology
Biopsy forceps   instruments which can be used to perform a biopsy
Blood count   measure of the number of erythrocytes, thrombocytes, platelets and leucocytes per cubic millimetre of blood (per litre of blood)
Blood pressure   pressure of blood against walls of blood vessels/heart
Blood sugar   amount of carbohydrate in the blood, measure of glucose level
Bradycardia   slow heartbeat
Bronchiectasis   bronchioles dilated due to obstruction
Bronchoscopy   examination, by visual inspection of the bronchus using a bronchoscope
Brook airway   instrument used for expired air resuscitation
Burn   injury by dry heat
Cachexia   wasting away of the body usually associated with malignant disease
Calculi   small mineral deposits usually found in the biliary or renal tract

Cannula hollow tube inserted into a body cavity for the introduction of substances

Cardiac arrest cessation of cardiac output

Carrier person who has micro-organisms without showing symptoms

Catheter tube for introduction of fluid into the body or the discharge of substances e.g. urine

Catheterisation insertion of a catheter

Cathetron unit remote controlled unit for placing radioactive cobalt into the cervix and uterus

Cautery instrument to coagulate blood vessels or destroy tissue by chemical means or heat

Cholelithiasis formation of gall stones

Cirrhosis fibrotic tissue replaces hepatic cells of the liver

Claustrophobia fear of confined spaces

Colic acute abdominal pain usually associated with biliary or renal calculi blocking a duct

Colonic washout method of clearing the bowel of faecal matter

Colostomy artificial anus on anterior abdominal wall

Coma unconsciousness from which the patient cannot be aroused

Comatose being in a coma

Comminuted fracture a break in the bone where the bone is fragmented

Complicated fracture a break in the bone with associated blood vessel or nerve injury

Compound dislocation joint dislocation where there is an external wound communicating with the joint

Compound fracture when part of the fracture is in contact with the external surface of the body

Compression band immobilisation device which also displaces body tissue laterally and therefore enables a reduction in radiographic exposure to be made

Compression bandage a bandage applied, over cotton wool pads, to joints to help to reduce infusion into the joint space

Concussion a state resulting from the brain being shaken violently

Contrast agent a drug introduced into the body for diagnostic purpose to outline a space or organ

Contusion injury by a blow when the skin is not broken e.g. a bruise

Cross-infection infection that a patient receives from another person

Cryosurgery destruction of diseased tissue by freezing, without harming adjacent tissue

Cyanosis a bluish tinge to the skin due to lack of oxygen

Cytotoxic drugs drugs which inhibit the growth of cells

Decubitus ulcer (pressure sore) ulcer due to lack of blood supply to a pressure area

Desquamation peeling of skin

Diabetic a person suffering from diabetes

Diabetic coma unconsciousness due to lack of insulin

Diarrhoea excess bowel motions

Diathermy use of heat to coagulate tissues

Disinfectant agent that destroys or inhibits the growth of micro-organisms but not necessarily spores

Dislocation displacement of one or more bones with relation to each other

Disposable items articles which are only used once and then discarded, reduces cross-infection

Diuresis increased excretion of urine

Diverticulitis pouches in the bowel which protrude through the bowel wall

Drug a substance used as a medicine

Dyspepsia disturbed digestion/indigestion

Dysphagia difficulty in swallowing

Dysphonia difficulty in speaking

Dyspnoea difficulty in breathing

Dystrophy degeneration

Dysuria painful or difficult urination

Embolism blood clot blocking a blood vessel

Emetic a drug used to induce vomiting

Enema a rectal injection of fluid

Epilation loss of hair

Epilepsy brain disorder which produces fits

Epileptic a person who suffers from epilepsy

Epistaxis nose bleed

Erythema redness of the skin

Filamented swab swab used in surgery with a radiopaque thread so it can be detected radiographically if necessary

Fistula an abnormal passage between two organs

Flatulence excessive gas in the stomach and intestinal tract

Fomite an article which carries pathogenic micro-organisms

Fracture a break in bone continuity

General anaesthesia   total loss of consciousness and therefore insensitivity to pain

Gram stain   — positive, organisms retain staining solution — negative, organisms lose staining solution and will take up counter stain

Greenstick fracture   incomplete break of the bone in young children

Haematemesis   vomiting of blood

Haematoma   a swelling due to a collection of blood

Haematuria   blood in the urine

Haemodialysis   treatment for renal failure

Haemoptysis   coughing up of blood

Haemorrhoids   collection of blood vessels at the anus — piles

Hemiplegia   paralysis of one side of the body

Histology   study of cells, organs and tissues

Hormone   chemical which acts on organs remote from its origin

Hyperglycaemic coma   (diabetic coma) excess of sugar in the blood causing loss of consciousness

Hyperpyrexia   high temperature over 40.6°C

Hypertension   high blood pressure

Hypertrophy   increase in size of an organ

Hypochondriac   person who thinks they are ill when they are not

Hypodermic   beneath the skin

Hypoglycaemic   low level of sugar in the blood

Hypotension   low blood pressure

Hypothermia   low body temperature below 35°C

Incision   clean cut which bleeds freely

Immunisation   introduction of antibodies to protect a person from disease

Impaction   when one aspect of a bone is growing into another. When one fragment of fractured bone is driven into another

Incontinence   inability to control the evacuation of faeces/urine

Infarction   area of necrotic tissue

Infection   invasion of a person or object by organisms e.g. bacteria

Inflammation   reaction of tissues to injury

Infusion   introduction of a liquid into the body over a long period of time

Injection   introducing a liquid into the body via a needle

Insomnia   sleeplessness

Insulin coma unconsciousness as a result of an overdose of insulin

Intravenous injection injection into a vein

Ischaemia diminished blood supply

Jaundice raised serum bilirubin causing yellowing of skin

Laceration 'torn' wound

Laryngeal mirror mirror for inspecting oral cavity and larynx

Laxative agent to relieve constipation

Leucoplakia white patches on mucous membrane, pre-malignant condition

Leukaemia cancer of the blood forming white cells

Leucocytosis increase in the total number of white blood cells

Leucopenia decrease in the number of leucocytes in the blood

Local anaesthetic a drug used to render a specific area of the body insensitive to pain

Malignant growth a growth which if not checked will spread locally, usually metastasise and eventually terminate in death

Mastectomy surgical removal of a breast

Medicine a substance used for treating disease

Menorrhagia excessive menstrual flow

Metastasis a secondary tumour produced by a malignant primary tumour

Myocardial infarction occlusion of a coronary artery

Necrosis death of tissue

Neoplasm new growth

Nephritis inflammation of the kidney

Neuralgia pain in a nerve

Neurosis abnormal anxiety

Obese overweight (excessive)

Oedema collection of lymph causing swelling

Opaque media contrast agents

Opaque medium contrast agent

Ophthalmoscope instrument for examining the interior of the eye

Osteoporosis deossification of bone

Osteosclerosis increased density of bone

Palliative relieves symptoms but does not cure

Paralysis loss of muscle function and sensation

Paraparesis partial paralysis of lower limbs

Paraplegic person with paralysis of the lower limbs

Parenteral outside the alimentary tract, injection through the skin

Pathogen   agent capable of producing disease
Pathological condition   condition caused by disease
Polyuria   passage of excessive quantities of urine
Post anaesthesia   after anaesthetic and before full recovery
Premedication   drug given prior to an anaesthetic to calm the
  patient
Pressure area   area where a decubitus ulcer may develop e.g.
  buttocks, elbows
Pressure point   place where a pulse is felt — where a
  superficial artery crosses a bone
Pressure sore   see decubitus ulcer
Proctitis   inflammation of the anus or rectum
Prolapse   the sinking down of an organ e.g. rectum, uterus
Prophylactic   agent which prevents the development of a disease
Prosthesis   artificial body part
Psoriasis   inflammation of skin, reddened areas with white scales
Pulmonary embolism   blockage of a blood vessel in the lungs
Pulse rate   number of cardiac contractions per minute
Purgative   a strong drug to encourage complete bowel evacuation
Pyrexia   fever
Respiratory rate   number of breaths per minute
Resuscitation   restoration of life after apparent death
Retention of urine   inability to pass urine
Reverse Barrier Nursing   special nursing procedure when a
  person is prone to infection
Rubor   redness due to inflammation
Scald   injury caused by moist heat
Scalpel   a surgical knife
Scoliosis   lateral curvature of the spine
Selection unit   remote controlled unit for placing radioactive
  caesium 137 into body cavities
Sedation   state induced by a drug to calm and allay pain
Shock   a condition when there is insufficient blood to fill the
  major arteries
Sinus   an abnormal passage opening on the skin surface
Sphygmomanometer   instrument for measuring blood pressure
Spina bifida   damage to vertebral arches
Spirometer   used to measure respiratory volumes and capacity
Sprain   tearing ligament or tissue in a joint
Stenosis   narrowing
Sterile   free from micro-organisms
Sterilisation   to render free from micro-organisms

Strain overstretching a muscle

Stupor when a person is partly conscious but can be roused

Subluxation partial dislocation

Suction apparatus for removing secretions

Surgical mask a mask to cover the nose and mouth to prevent the contamination of a sterile area by droplet infection

Symptoms an indication of a particular disorder of which the patient complains

Syndrome a group of symptoms which characterise a disease or lesion

Syringe instrument for holding fluid for injection

Tachycardia rapid heart beat

Thrombosis clot in a vessel

Tinnitus ringing in the ears

Tracheostomy artificial opening in the trachea or insertion of a tube, to maintain breathing

Ulcer open sore, cause inflammatory process breaking through skin

Unconscious a lack of awareness, with no reflexes

Uraemia excessive urea in blood, cause renal failure

Urinal a vessel for receiving urine

Urinary catheter catheter inserted into the urinary bladder to drain urine

Urticaria raised red or white weals on the skin

Venous haemorrhage bleeding from a vein

Vertigo feeling of loss of balance

Vesico-ureteric reflux urine passes from bladder to ureter

Virus smaller than bacterium, with little sensitivity to antibiotics

Vomit bowl receptacle to receive vomit

Index